The Alzheimer's diet cookbook for beginners 2024

A Flavorful Journey through The Alzheimer's Diet Cookbook for Beginners

John B. Alcock

Table of Contents

INTRODUCTION..**11**

What is Alzheimer's Disease?.................................**11**

The Impact of Nutrition on Alzheimer's................**13**

2. Effects on Neurodegeneration:..........................**14**

CHAPTER ONE **17**

BASICS OF ALZHEIMER'S DIET...............**17**

Nutritional Guidelines for Alzheimer's **17**

Importance of a Balanced Diet...............................**20**

Key Nutrients for Brain Health..............................**24**

CHAPTER TWO **29**

GETTING STARTED ON ALZHEIMER DIET29

Setting Up an Alzheimer's-Friendly Kitchen........**29**

Essential Kitchen Tools..**32**

Stocking Alzheimer's-Friendly Ingredients..........**37**

CHAPTER THREE **40**

BREAKFAST RECIPES....................................**40**

Berry Blast Smoothie Bowl **40**

Avocado and Tomato Breakfast Toast..................**42**

Cinnamon Apple Oatmeal **43**

Spinach and Feta Egg Muffins 44

Chia Seed Pudding with Mixed Berries 46

Banana and Almond Butter Stuffed French Toast 47

Yogurt Parfait with Granola and Berries 49

Vegetable and Cheese Omelette 50

Quinoa and Fruit Salad 51

Pumpkin Spice Overnight Oats............................53

Broccoli and Cheese Egg Muffins 54

Mango and Coconut Chia Pudding.....................56

Turkey and Vegetable Breakfast Wrap 57

Blueberry Almond Oat Bars 58

Peach and Walnut Breakfast Quinoa...................61

Pumpkin Pancakes with Maple Syrup 62

Smoked Salmon and Avocado Bagel 63

Coconut Banana Baked Oatmeal.......................64

Spinach and Mushroom Breakfast Quesadilla 66

CHAPTER FOUR..................................**68**

LUNCH RECIPES **68**

Salmon and Quinoa Salad.........................68

Vegetarian Lentil Soup 69

Chicken and Vegetable Stir-Fry 70

Sweet Potato and Black Bean Buddha Bowl 72

Turkey and Cranberry Wrap 73

Caprese Salad with Grilled Chicken 75

Mushroom and Spinach Quiche 76

Eggplant and Tomato Stuffed Bell Peppers.........79

Shrimp and Avocado Salad..................................80

Quinoa and Vegetable Stir-Fry............................82

Mediterranean Chickpea Salad 83

Salmon and Asparagus Foil Packets 84

Vegetable and Turkey Wrap 86

Lentil and Spinach Curry.....................................87

Shrimp and Vegetable Skewers 89

Turkey and Vegetable Stir-Fried Brown Rice......90

Chickpea and Vegetable Stew.............................91

Turkey and Vegetable Brown Rice Bowl..............93

Egg Salad Lettuce Wraps 94

CHAPTER FIVE 97

DINNER RECIPES................................97

Baked Lemon Herb Chicken 97

Vegetarian Stuffed Bell Peppers 98

Salmon and Sweet Potato Foil Packets 99

Turkey and Vegetable Skillet.................................101

Cauliflower Fried Rice with Shrimp 102

Mushroom and Spinach Stuffed Chicken Breast....104

Vegetable and Lentil Curry...................................105

Pesto Zoodles with Grilled Chicken.......................107

Baked Cod with Lemon Dill Sauce 108

Chickpea and Vegetable Stir-Fry 109

Eggplant Parmesan...112

Salmon and Spinach Stuffed Portobello Mushrooms
....114

Vegetarian Chickpea and Sweet Potato Curry.......115

Teriyaki Chicken Stir-Fry......................................116

Quinoa and Black Bean Stuffed Peppers...............118

Lemon Garlic Shrimp and Broccoli Pasta..............119

Baked Herb-Crusted Cod......................................121

Vegetable and Chickpea Stir-Fry 122

Mango Glazed Chicken Skewers 124

CHAPTER SIX **126**

SNACKS AND APPETIZERS **126**

Chia Seed Pudding Parfait...............................126

Sweet Potato and Rosemary Bites...................127

Cottage Cheese Stuffed Strawberries...................128

Mango Salsa with Cucumber Chips 129

Edamame and Mint Hummus...................131

Tomato Basil Bruschetta 132

Almond Butter and Banana Bites 133

Pumpkin Seeds and Cranberry Mix...................134

Caprese Skewers...................135

Guacamole-Stuffed Cucumber Cups 136

Quinoa and Vegetable Stuffed Bell Peppers...................138

Smoked Salmon Cucumber Bites 139

Roasted Chickpeas 141

Zucchini and Goat Cheese Roll-Ups...................142

Mushroom and Spinach Stuffed Phyllo Cups...................143

Tuna Salad Lettuce Wraps...................145

Cauliflower Buffalo Bites 146

Egg Salad Stuffed Cucumber Cups 147

Sesame Ginger Snap Peas............................149

Peach and Goat Cheese Crostini............................150

CHAPTER SEVEN **152**

DESSERTS WITH BENEFITS........................**152**

Berry Yogurt Parfait............................152

Avocado Chocolate Mousse............................153

Chia Seed and Mango Pudding 154

Banana-Oat Cookies............................156

Coconut and Berry Chia Popsicles............................157

Apple and Almond Butter Nachos 159

Pumpkin Spice Energy Balls 160

Almond and Blueberry Frozen Yogurt Bites 161

Cinnamon Baked Pears 163

Dark Chocolate-Dipped Strawberries............................164

Turmeric Golden Milk Popsicles............................166

Matcha Green Tea Chia Pudding............................167

Papaya and Lime Sorbet............................169

Walnut and Date Energy Bites 170

Blueberry and Almond Flour Mug Cake 171

Cocoa Avocado Pudding............................173

Raspberry and Almond Tartlets 174

Coconut and Pineapple Chia Seed Popsicles 176

Mango and Coconut Rice Pudding 178

CHAPTER EIGHT **181**

MEAL PLAN **181**

Day 1 181

Day 2 181

Day 3 181

Day 4 182

Day 5 182

Day 6 182

Day 7 183

Day 8 183

Day 9 184

Day 10 184

Day 11 184

Day 12 185

Day 13 185

Day 14 185

Day 15 186

Day 16...186

Day 17...187

Day 18...187

Day 19...187

Day 20...188

Day 21...188

Conclusion...................................189

INTRODUCTION

What is Alzheimer's Disease?

Alzheimer's disease is a progressive neurodegenerative disorder that primarily affects the brain, leading to a decline in cognitive function and memory. It is the most common cause of dementia, a syndrome characterized by a significant loss of cognitive abilities that interfere with daily life. Alzheimer's disease gets its name from Dr. Alois Alzheimer, a German physician who first described the condition in 1906.

Key Features of Alzheimer's Disease:

- ***Neuronal Damage:*** Alzheimer's disease involves the gradual damage and death of nerve cells (neurons) in the brain, particularly in regions responsible for memory and cognitive functions.

- ***Formation of Amyloid Plaques and Tau Tangles:*** Abnormal protein aggregates called amyloid plaques and tau tangles build up in the brain. These deposits disrupt the normal functioning of neurons and are considered hallmark characteristics of Alzheimer's.

- ***Progressive Cognitive Decline:*** The disease progresses over time, leading to a decline in cognitive abilities such as memory, reasoning, language skills, and problem-solving. Individuals may also experience changes in behavior and personality.

- **Stages of Alzheimer's:** Alzheimer's disease typically advances through stages, from mild cognitive impairment (MCI) to more severe stages where individuals may lose the ability to carry out daily activities.

- **Aging and Genetic Factors:** While age is a significant risk factor for Alzheimer's, genetic factors also play a role. Certain genetic mutations are associated with a higher risk of developing the disease, though they are not deterministic.

- **Diagnosis and Assessment:** Diagnosis is often based on a combination of clinical assessments, medical history, cognitive testing, and sometimes brain imaging. Early diagnosis is crucial for implementing interventions that may slow down the progression of symptoms.

- **No Cure, but Management Strategies:** Currently, there is no cure for Alzheimer's disease. Treatment focuses on managing symptoms, improving quality of life, and providing support for individuals and their caregivers.

- ***Global Impact:*** Alzheimer's disease has a significant societal impact, affecting millions of people worldwide. It poses challenges not only for individuals living with the disease but also for their families, caregivers, and healthcare systems.

The Impact of Nutrition on Alzheimer's

The impact of nutrition on Alzheimer's disease is profound, with emerging evidence suggesting that diet plays a crucial role in the prevention and management of the condition. Here's an overview of how nutrition influences Alzheimer's:

1. Brain Health and Nutrients:

- ***Essential Nutrients:*** Certain nutrients are vital for maintaining brain health and cognitive function. These include omega-3 fatty acids, antioxidants (such as vitamins C and E), B vitamins (especially B6, B12, and folate), and minerals like zinc and magnesium.

- ***Anti-inflammatory Foods:*** Chronic inflammation in the brain is believed to contribute to Alzheimer's disease progression. Consuming anti-inflammatory foods, such as fruits, vegetables, nuts, and fatty fish, may help mitigate inflammation and protect against cognitive decline.

2. Effects on Neurodegeneration:

- ***Role of Oxidative Stress:*** Oxidative stress, caused by an imbalance between antioxidants and free radicals in the body, is implicated in the development of Alzheimer's disease. Antioxidant-rich foods can help neutralize free radicals and reduce oxidative damage to brain cells.

- ***Neuroprotective Properties:*** Certain compounds found in plant-based foods, such as flavonoids and polyphenols, have neuroprotective properties and may help preserve cognitive function. These compounds are abundant in fruits, vegetables, tea, and red wine.

3. Influence on Risk Factors:

- ***Heart-Healthy Diet:*** Many dietary patterns associated with a reduced risk of cardiovascular disease, such as the Mediterranean diet and the DASH (Dietary Approaches to Stop Hypertension) diet, have also been linked to a lower risk of Alzheimer's disease. These diets emphasize whole grains, lean proteins, healthy fats, and plenty of fruits and vegetables.

- ***Blood Sugar Regulation:*** Emerging research suggests that maintaining stable blood sugar levels may be important for brain health and Alzheimer's prevention. Diets high in refined sugars and carbohydrates may increase the risk of cognitive decline, while diets rich in fiber, whole grains, and healthy fats can help stabilize blood sugar levels.

4. Potential Therapeutic Benefits:

- ***Nutritional Interventions:*** Some studies suggest that specific dietary interventions, such as the ketogenic diet or dietary supplementation with certain nutrients (e.g., curcumin, resveratrol), may have therapeutic potential in Alzheimer's disease. However, more research is needed to confirm their efficacy and safety.

- ***Personalized Nutrition:*** Individual factors such as genetics, metabolism, and gut microbiota may influence how diet impacts Alzheimer's risk and progression. Personalized nutrition approaches tailored to an individual's unique characteristics may hold promise for optimizing brain health.

5. Lifestyle Factors:

- **_Combined Approach:_** While nutrition plays a crucial role, it is just one aspect of a comprehensive approach to Alzheimer's prevention and management. Regular physical exercise, mental stimulation, adequate sleep, stress management, and social engagement are also essential for maintaining cognitive vitality and overall well-being.

CHAPTER ONE

BASICS OF ALZHEIMER'S DIET

Nutritional Guidelines for Alzheimer's

Nutritional guidelines for Alzheimer's aim to support overall health, cognitive function, and quality of life. While there is no one-size-fits-all approach, the following general recommendations can be beneficial for individuals with Alzheimer's disease:

Balanced Diet:

- Emphasize a balanced diet that includes a variety of nutrient-dense foods from all food groups.
- Prioritize fruits, vegetables, whole grains, lean proteins, and healthy fats.

Omega-3 Fatty Acids:

- Include sources of omega-3 fatty acids, such as fatty fish (salmon, trout, sardines), walnuts, flaxseeds, and chia seeds.
- Omega-3s are believed to have neuroprotective properties and may support brain health.

Antioxidant-Rich Foods:

- Consume a variety of fruits and vegetables rich in antioxidants, including berries, leafy greens, and colorful vegetables.
- Antioxidants help combat oxidative stress, which is associated with cognitive decline.

Healthy Fats:

- Choose sources of healthy fats, such as olive oil, avocados, nuts, and seeds.
- Limit saturated and trans fats found in processed and fried foods.

Adequate Hydration:

- Ensure proper hydration by drinking an adequate amount of water throughout the day.
- Dehydration can contribute to confusion and cognitive impairment.

Whole Grains:

- Opt for whole grains like brown rice, quinoa, and whole wheat bread over refined grains.
- Whole grains provide sustained energy and essential nutrients.

Lean Proteins:

- Include lean protein sources, such as poultry, fish, legumes, and tofu.

- Protein is important for muscle maintenance and overall health.

Moderate Sugar and Refined Carbohydrates:

- Limit the intake of added sugars and refined carbohydrates.
- High sugar consumption may contribute to inflammation and cognitive decline.

Vitamin and Mineral Supplementation:

- Consult with a healthcare professional about the need for vitamin and mineral supplements.
- Adequate levels of vitamins B, C, D, and E, as well as minerals like zinc and magnesium, are important for cognitive health.

Regular and Consistent Meals:

- Establish a routine with regular and consistent mealtimes.
- Structure and routine can be beneficial for individuals with Alzheimer's.

Adapt Textures and Presentation:

- Modify food textures as needed, especially if there are swallowing difficulties.
- Present visually appealing and easily recognizable foods to encourage eating.

Consider Individual Preferences:

- Take into account individual preferences, cultural considerations, and dietary restrictions.
- Adapt the diet to suit personal tastes while still meeting nutritional needs.

Monitor for Weight Changes:

- Regularly monitor weight and nutritional status.
- Address any unintended weight loss or gain with the guidance of healthcare professionals.

Collaborate with Healthcare Providers:

- Collaborate with healthcare providers, including dietitians and nutritionists, to tailor dietary recommendations to individual needs.
- Consideration of medications and potential interactions is crucial.

Importance of a Balanced Diet

A balanced diet is crucial for maintaining overall health and well-being. It provides the body with the necessary nutrients in the right proportions, supporting various physiological functions and preventing the risk of nutritional deficiencies. Here are several reasons highlighting the importance of a balanced diet:

Nutrient Adequacy:

- A balanced diet ensures an adequate intake of essential nutrients such as vitamins, minerals, proteins, carbohydrates, and fats.
- Each nutrient plays a specific role in maintaining health, supporting growth and development, and preventing various diseases.

Energy for Daily Activities:

- Carbohydrates, proteins, and fats from a balanced diet provide the body with the energy required for daily activities, including work, exercise, and cognitive functions.
- Balancing macronutrients helps maintain stable energy levels throughout the day.

Weight Management:

- A balanced diet helps in managing body weight by providing the right combination of nutrients without excess calories.
- Proper nutrition supports a healthy metabolism and reduces the risk of obesity-related conditions.

Supports Growth and Development:

- In children, adolescents, and pregnant women, a balanced diet is essential for proper growth and development.

- Nutrients like calcium, vitamin D, and protein are crucial for bone health and muscle development.

Disease Prevention:

- A well-balanced diet is associated with a lower risk of chronic diseases such as heart disease, diabetes, and certain types of cancer.

- Antioxidants and anti-inflammatory compounds found in fruits and vegetables contribute to overall health and disease prevention.

Optimal Organ Function:

- Nutrients support the optimal function of various organs, including the heart, brain, liver, kidneys, and immune system.

- A balanced diet contributes to the maintenance of healthy blood pressure, cholesterol levels, and overall cardiovascular health.

Digestive Health:

- Dietary fiber from whole grains, fruits, and vegetables aids in digestion and helps prevent constipation.

- Adequate water intake, along with fiber, supports a healthy digestive system.

Mental Health and Cognitive Function:

- Proper nutrition is linked to cognitive function and mental well-being.
- Omega-3 fatty acids, found in fish and certain nuts, have been associated with improved cognitive function and mood.

Hormonal Balance:

- Balanced nutrition contributes to the regulation of hormonal levels in the body.
- Proper hormone balance is crucial for reproductive health, metabolism, and overall physiological function.

Immune System Support:

- Nutrients such as vitamins A, C, D, and zinc play a role in supporting the immune system.
- A balanced diet contributes to the body's ability to fight off infections and illnesses.

Long-Term Health and Longevity:

- Adopting a balanced diet is a key component of a healthy lifestyle that can contribute to overall longevity and well-being.

- Consistent adherence to a balanced diet is associated with a higher quality of life in the long term.

Key Nutrients for Brain Health

Maintaining optimal brain health requires a combination of essential nutrients that support cognitive function, protect against oxidative stress, and promote overall neurological well-being. Here are key nutrients crucial for brain health:

Omega-3 Fatty Acids:

- ***Sources:*** Fatty fish (salmon, trout, sardines), flaxseeds, chia seeds, walnuts.
- ***Benefits:*** Omega-3 fatty acids, especially EPA and DHA, are integral components of cell membranes in the brain, supporting communication between brain cells and reducing inflammation.

Antioxidants (Vitamins C and E):

- ***Sources:*** Citrus fruits, berries, spinach, almonds, sunflower seeds.
- ***Benefits:*** Antioxidants protect brain cells from oxidative stress, which is linked to cognitive

decline. They neutralize free radicals that can cause cellular damage.

B Vitamins (B6, B12, Folate):

- *Sources:* Whole grains, lean meats, poultry, fish, eggs, dairy products, leafy greens.

- *Benefits:* B vitamins play a crucial role in the production of neurotransmitters, including serotonin and dopamine. They are essential for cognitive function and may help reduce the risk of age-related cognitive decline.

Vitamin D:

- *Sources:* Fatty fish, fortified dairy products, eggs, exposure to sunlight.

- *Benefits:* Vitamin D is important for brain development and function. Low levels of vitamin D have been associated with an increased risk of cognitive impairment.

Iron:

- *Sources:* Lean meats, poultry, fish, beans, lentils, fortified cereals.

- *Benefits:* Iron is vital for the production of hemoglobin, which transports oxygen to the brain.

Iron deficiency may lead to cognitive issues and difficulty concentrating.

Zinc:

- ***Sources:*** Meat, dairy products, nuts, seeds, whole grains.
- ***Benefits:*** Zinc is involved in neurotransmitter function and may play a role in memory and learning. It also has antioxidant properties.

Magnesium:

- ***Sources:*** Leafy greens, nuts, seeds, whole grains, legumes.
- ***Benefits:*** Magnesium supports synaptic plasticity, the ability of the brain to change and adapt. It may also have a calming effect on the nervous system.

Choline:

- ***Sources:*** Eggs, liver, soy products, cruciferous vegetables.
- ***Benefits:*** Choline is a precursor to acetylcholine, a neurotransmitter important for memory and mood regulation. It is crucial for cognitive development.

Phosphatidylserine:

- ***Sources:*** Fish, organ meats, soybeans.

- **Benefits:** Phosphatidylserine is a component of cell membranes and plays a role in cell signaling. It may support cognitive function and memory.

Curcumin (Turmeric):

- **Sources:** Turmeric, a spice commonly used in curry dishes.
- **Benefits:** Curcumin has anti-inflammatory and antioxidant properties. It may contribute to neuroprotection and support cognitive function.

Flavonoids:

- **Sources:** Berries, citrus fruits, tea, dark chocolate.
- **Benefits:** Flavonoids have antioxidant and anti-inflammatory effects, potentially protecting against cognitive decline and promoting brain health.

Protein:

- **Sources:** Lean meats, poultry, fish, dairy products, legumes, tofu.
- **Benefits:** Proteins provide amino acids, the building blocks for neurotransmitters. They support overall brain function and repair.

Folate:

- **Sources:** Leafy greens, legumes, fortified cereals.

- ***Benefits:*** Folate is essential for DNA synthesis and repair. It plays a role in cognitive function and may help reduce the risk of age-related cognitive decline.

Coenzyme Q10 (CoQ10):

- ***Sources:*** Fatty fish, organ meats, whole grains, nuts.
- ***Benefits:*** CoQ10 is an antioxidant that supports mitochondrial function, enhancing energy production in brain cells.

Probiotics:

- ***Sources:*** Yogurt, kefir, fermented foods (kimchi, sauerkraut).
- ***Benefits:*** Gut health is linked to brain health. Probiotics support a healthy gut microbiome, which may influence cognitive function and mood.

CHAPTER TWO

GETTING STARTED ON ALZHEIMER DIET

Setting Up an Alzheimer's-Friendly Kitchen

Setting up an Alzheimer's-friendly kitchen involves creating an environment that supports the needs and abilities of individuals living with Alzheimer's disease. This includes considerations for safety, simplicity, and ease of use. Here are some tips for setting up an Alzheimer's-friendly kitchen:

Clear and Accessible Layout:

- ***Minimize Clutter:*** Keep countertops clear of unnecessary items to reduce visual confusion.
- ***Organize Essentials:*** Arrange commonly used items within easy reach to minimize frustration.

Safe Cooking Spaces:

- ***Secure Appliances:*** Ensure that appliances are safely secured to countertops to prevent accidental spills or falls.
- ***Safety Features:*** Consider appliances with safety features such as automatic shut-off.

Easy-to-Use Utensils and Tools:

- ***Ergonomic Utensils:*** Provide utensils with easy grips and ergonomic handles for comfortable use.
- ***Color Contrast:*** Use utensils with contrasting colors to make them easily distinguishable.

Labeling and Identification:

- ***Clear Labels:*** Label drawers, cabinets, and containers with clear and simple labels or pictures.
- ***Color-Coded System:*** Use a color-coded system to help identify different items or areas in the kitchen.

Simple and Safe Cookware:

- ***Non-Slip Mats:*** Place non-slip mats under rugs and at key locations to prevent slipping.
- ***Safe Cookware:*** Choose cookware with safety features, such as cool-touch handles.

Accessible Storage:

- ***Lower Shelves:*** Store frequently used items on lower shelves for easy access.
- ***Visible Storage:*** Use clear containers for easy visibility of stored items.

Kitchen Safety Measures:

- ***Emergency Information:*** Keep emergency contact information and important instructions visible.
- ***Fire Safety:*** Install smoke detectors and ensure that fire extinguishers are easily accessible.

Simple Recipes and Instructions:

- ***Clear Instructions:*** Use simple, step-by-step instructions for cooking and meal preparation.
- ***Visual Aids:*** Include visual aids or pictures to assist with understanding.

Routine and Consistency:

- ***Establish Routine:*** Stick to a consistent mealtime routine to provide a sense of structure.
- ***Familiar Layout:*** Keep the kitchen layout consistent to reduce confusion.

Assistance and Supervision:

- ***Caregiver Support:*** Have a caregiver or support person available if additional assistance is needed.
- ***Supervised Cooking:*** Supervise cooking activities to ensure safety and prevent accidents.

Nutritional Convenience:

- ***Prepared Ingredients:*** Consider using pre-chopped or pre-prepared ingredients for convenience.
- ***Healthy Snacks:*** Keep nutritious snacks readily available for quick and accessible options.

Comfortable Seating:

- ***Chair or Stool:*** Provide a comfortable chair or stool for breaks during meal preparation.
- ***Accessible Seating:*** Ensure that seating is easily accessible for individuals with mobility challenges.

Natural Lighting:

- ***Maximize Natural Light:*** Increase natural lighting in the kitchen to enhance visibility.
- ***Well-Lit Areas:*** Install additional lighting in key areas for safety.

Regular Maintenance:

- ***Check Appliances:*** Regularly inspect and maintain kitchen appliances to ensure they are in good working condition.
- ***Adjust as Needed:*** Be flexible and make adjustments to the kitchen setup based on the individual's evolving needs

Essential Kitchen Tools

Creating an Alzheimer's-friendly kitchen involves organizing the space and selecting tools that enhance safety, accessibility, and ease of use. Here is a list of essential kitchen tools to consider:

Non-Slip Flooring:

- Use slip-resistant flooring or place non-slip rugs or mats in areas where water or spills are common.

Clear Pathways:

- Ensure clear pathways in the kitchen to minimize the risk of tripping or bumping into objects.

Task Lighting:

- Install bright task lighting under cabinets and in work areas to improve visibility and reduce shadows.

Contrasting Colors:

- Choose contrasting colors for countertops, utensils, and cutting boards to enhance visibility and reduce confusion.

Labeling:

- Label drawers, cabinets, and containers with large, clear labels to help identify contents easily.

Easy-Grip Utensils:

- Opt for utensils with ergonomic handles or those designed for easy gripping.
- Consider adaptive utensils with larger handles or built-up grips for better control.

One-Handed Cutting Board:

- Choose a cutting board with non-slip edges or a built-in knife guide to make chopping safer and easier.

Electric Can Opener:

- Use an electric can opener for easier and safer can opening.
- Look for models with large, easy-to-press buttons.

Automatic Shut-Off Appliances:

- Choose appliances, such as kettles and toasters, with automatic shut-off features for safety.

Microwave with Simple Controls:

- Select a microwave with easy-to-read and simple controls.
- Use labels or markers to highlight essential buttons.

Color-Coded Cookware:

- Use color-coded cookware for easy identification and to match with corresponding utensils.
- Consider non-stick pans for easier cooking and cleaning.

Large, Visible Timer:

- Provide a large, easy-to-read timer to assist with monitoring cooking times.
- Choose timers with audible alarms.

Organized Storage:

- Arrange frequently used items at eye level for easy access.
- Use clear containers for storing ingredients to enhance visibility.

Non-Skid Bowls and Plates:

- Choose bowls and plates with non-skid bases to prevent accidental spills.

- Consider weighted or suction-based dinnerware for added stability.

Simple Menu Boards:

- Display a simple menu board or chart with meal options and steps for meal preparation.

Easy-to-Read Thermostats:

- Install easy-to-read thermostats on ovens and stovetops.
- Consider appliances with safety features like automatic shut-off.

Accessible Shelving:

- Ensure that frequently used items are stored in easily accessible shelves or drawers.

Faucet with Temperature Control:

- Install faucets with easy-to-use temperature controls to prevent burns.

Automatic Shut-Off Appliances:

- Consider appliances, such as kettles and toasters, with automatic shut-off features for safety.

Assistive Devices:

- Explore assistive devices like jar openers, easy-grip peelers, and adaptive cutting tools to simplify tasks.

Emergency Information:

- Keep emergency contact information and instructions for appliance use visible in the kitchen.

Comfortable Seating:

- Provide comfortable and stable seating in the kitchen for breaks and meal preparation.

Phone Access:

- Ensure easy access to a phone in case of emergencies

Stocking Alzheimer's-Friendly Ingredients

Easy-to-Identify Foods:

- Choose foods with clear packaging and recognizable labels.

- Organize ingredients in labeled, transparent containers.

Pre-Cut and Prepped Items:

- Opt for pre-cut fruits, vegetables, and meats to save preparation time.
- Consider frozen pre-portioned meals for convenience.

Healthy Snack Options:

- Stock up on nutritious and easy-to-eat snacks like nuts, yogurt, and cut-up fruits.
- Provide accessible snack stations with portioned options.

Hydration Choices:

- Keep a variety of hydrating options like water, herbal teas, and low-sugar juices.
- Use labeled cups or bottles for easy recognition.

Whole Grains and Fiber:

- Include whole grains such as brown rice, quinoa, and whole-grain bread.
- Offer high-fiber options like oats, legumes, and whole fruits.

Protein-Rich Foods:

- Ensure a variety of protein sources like lean meats, poultry, fish, and plant-based proteins.
- Include protein-rich snacks such as Greek yogurt and cheese.

Dairy and Dairy Alternatives:

- Provide dairy or fortified dairy alternatives for calcium and vitamin D.
- Choose options with clear labeling and recognizable packaging.

Healthy Fats:

- Include sources of healthy fats like olive oil, avocados, and nuts.
- Offer pre-portioned options to maintain a balanced diet.

Adaptive Cooking Ingredients:

- Consider ready-to-use sauces, spices, and seasonings to simplify cooking.
- Pre-mix ingredients for common recipes to streamline the cooking process.

Comfort Foods and Favorites:

- Keep familiar and favorite foods to promote appetite and enjoyment.

- Include a variety of flavors and textures to cater to individual preferences.

CHAPTER THREE

BREAKFAST RECIPES

Berry Blast Smoothie Bowl

Ingredients:

- 1 cup mixed berries (blueberries, strawberries, raspberries)

- 1 banana, frozen

- 1/2 cup Greek yogurt

- 1 tablespoon chia seeds

- 1/4 cup almond milk

Preparation Time: 5 minutes

Cooking Time: N/A

Serving Time: 10 minutes

Nutritional Info:

- Calories: 250

- Protein: 10g

- Fiber: 8g

- Healthy Fats: 7g

Instructions:

- Blend the berries, frozen banana, Greek yogurt, chia seeds, and almond milk until smooth.

- Pour the smoothie into a bowl.

- Top with additional berries, sliced banana, and a sprinkle of chia seeds.

- Serve chilled.

Serving Methods:

1. Garnish with granola or nuts for added texture.

2. Drizzle honey or maple syrup for extra sweetness.

Avocado and Tomato Breakfast Toast

Ingredients:

- 1 slice whole-grain bread

- 1/2 ripe avocado, mashed

- Cherry tomatoes, sliced

- Salt and pepper to taste

- Fresh basil leaves for garnish

Preparation Time: 5 minutes

Cooking Time: 5 minutes

Serving Time: 10 minutes

Nutritional Info:

- Calories: 200

- Protein: 5g

- Fiber: 7g

- Healthy Fats: 10g

Instructions:

- Toast the whole-grain bread slice.

- Spread the mashed avocado evenly on the toast.

- Top with sliced cherry tomatoes.

- Season with salt and pepper and garnish with fresh basil leaves.

Serving Methods:

1. Drizzle with olive oil or balsamic glaze.

2. Serve with a poached or fried egg for added protein.

Cinnamon Apple Oatmeal

Ingredients:

- 1/2 cup old-fashioned oats

- 1 cup unsweetened almond milk

- 1 apple, peeled and diced

- 1/2 teaspoon ground cinnamon

- 1 tablespoon honey or maple syrup

Preparation Time: 5 minutes

Cooking Time: 10 minutes

Serving Time: 15 minutes

Nutritional Info:

- Calories: 300

- Protein: 6g

- Fiber: 8g

- Healthy Fats: 5g

Instructions:

- In a saucepan, combine oats and almond milk. Cook over medium heat.

- Add diced apples and cinnamon. Stir frequently until the oats are cooked and the apples are tender.

- Sweeten with honey or maple syrup.

- Serve warm.

Serving Methods:

1. Top with a dollop of Greek yogurt.

2. Sprinkle chopped nuts or seeds for added crunch.

Spinach and Feta Egg Muffins

Ingredients:

- 4 large eggs

- 1 cup fresh spinach, chopped

- 1/2 cup feta cheese, crumbled

- 1/4 cup red bell pepper, diced

- Salt and pepper to taste

Preparation Time: 10 minutes

Cooking Time: 15 minutes

Serving Time: 25 minutes

Nutritional Info:

- Calories: 220

- Protein: 15g

- Fiber: 2g

- Healthy Fats: 15g

Instructions:

- Preheat the oven to 350°F (175°C). Grease a muffin tin.

- In a bowl, whisk the eggs and season with salt and pepper.

- Stir in chopped spinach, feta cheese, and diced red bell pepper.

- Pour the mixture into the muffin cups and bake until the eggs are set.

- Allow to cool slightly before serving.

Serving Methods:

1. Serve with a side of whole-grain toast or a small fruit salad.

2. Drizzle with hot sauce or salsa for added flavor.

Chia Seed Pudding with Mixed Berries

Ingredients:

- 2 tablespoons chia seeds

- 1/2 cup almond milk

- 1/2 teaspoon vanilla extract

- Mixed berries for topping

Preparation Time: 5 minutes (plus overnight chilling)

Cooking Time: N/A

Serving Time: 10 minutes

Nutritional Info:

- Calories: 180

- Protein: 4g

- Fiber: 10g

- Healthy Fats: 8g

Instructions:

- In a bowl, mix chia seeds, almond milk, and vanilla extract.

- Stir well and refrigerate overnight or for at least 4 hours until the mixture thickens.

- Spoon the chia pudding into a serving dish and top with mixed berries.

Serving Methods:

1. Add a dollop of Greek yogurt or coconut yogurt.

2. Sprinkle with a teaspoon of crushed nuts or seeds.

Banana and Almond Butter Stuffed French Toast

Ingredients:

- 2 slices whole-grain bread

- 1 ripe banana, sliced

- 2 tablespoons almond butter

- 1 egg

- 1/4 cup almond milk

- 1/2 teaspoon cinnamon

Preparation Time: 10 minutes

Cooking Time: 10 minutes

Serving Time: 20 minutes

Nutritional Info:

- Calories: 350

- Protein: 12g

- Fiber: 6g

- Healthy Fats: 15g

Instructions:

- Spread almond butter on one side of each bread slice and place banana slices between them.

- In a bowl, whisk together the egg, almond milk, and cinnamon.

- Dip the stuffed bread slices into the egg mixture, coating both sides.

- Cook on a griddle or skillet until golden brown on each side.

Serving Methods:

- Top with a drizzle of honey or maple syrup.

- Garnish with additional banana slices and a sprinkle of cinnamon.

Yogurt Parfait with Granola and Berries

Ingredients:

- 1 cup Greek yogurt

- 1/4 cup granola

- Mixed berries (strawberries, blueberries)

- 1 tablespoon honey

Preparation Time: 5 minutes

Cooking Time: N/A

Serving Time: 10 minutes

Nutritional Info:

- Calories: 250

- Protein: 15g

- Fiber: 3g

- Healthy Fats: 7g

Instructions:

- In a glass or bowl, layer Greek yogurt with granola and mixed berries.

- Repeat the layers until the container is filled.

- Drizzle honey on top for sweetness.

- Serve immediately.

Serving Methods:

1. Substitute granola with chopped nuts or seeds.

2. Add a sprinkle of cinnamon for extra flavor.

Vegetable and Cheese Omelette

Ingredients:

- 2 eggs

- 1/4 cup bell peppers, diced

- 1/4 cup tomatoes, diced

- 2 tablespoons feta cheese, crumbled

- Fresh herbs (parsley, chives)

- Salt and pepper to taste

Preparation Time: 10 minutes

Cooking Time: 5 minutes

Serving Time: 15 minutes

Nutritional Info:

- Calories: 220

- Protein: 15g

- Fiber: 2g

- Healthy Fats: 15g

Instructions:

- Whisk eggs in a bowl and season with salt and pepper.

- In a non-stick skillet, sauté bell peppers and tomatoes until softened.

- Pour whisked eggs over the vegetables and cook until set.

- Sprinkle feta cheese and fresh herbs on one half of the omelette.

- Fold the omelette in half and slide onto a plate.

Serving Methods:

1. Serve with a side of whole-grain toast or a small green salad.

2. Top with a dollop of salsa or Greek yogurt.

Quinoa and Fruit Salad

Ingredients:

- 1/2 cup cooked quinoa

- 1/2 cup mixed fruit (pineapple, mango, kiwi)

- 2 tablespoons Greek yogurt

- 1 tablespoon honey

- Fresh mint leaves for garnish

Preparation Time: 15 minutes

Cooking Time: 15 minutes (for quinoa)

Serving Time: 30 minutes

Nutritional Info:

- Calories: 280

- Protein: 7g

- Fiber: 5g

- Healthy Fats: 3g

Instructions:

- In a bowl, combine cooked quinoa and mixed fruit.

- In a separate bowl, mix Greek yogurt and honey.

- Pour the yogurt mixture over the quinoa and fruit.

- Toss gently to coat, garnish with fresh mint leaves, and refrigerate for 15 minutes.

Serving Methods:

1. Top with a sprinkle of nuts or seeds for added crunch.

2. Serve in a hollowed-out melon for a creative presentation.

Pumpkin Spice Overnight Oats

Ingredients:

- 1/2 cup rolled oats

- 1/2 cup pumpkin puree

- 1/2 cup milk (dairy or plant-based)

- 1 tablespoon maple syrup

- 1/2 teaspoon pumpkin spice

- Chopped nuts for topping

Preparation Time: 5 minutes (plus overnight chilling)

Cooking Time: N/A

Serving Time: 10 minutes

Nutritional Info:

- Calories: 280

- Protein: 9g

- Fiber: 8g

- Healthy Fats: 6g

Instructions:

- In a jar, combine rolled oats, pumpkin puree, milk, maple syrup, and pumpkin spice.

- Stir well, cover, and refrigerate overnight.

- In the morning, give it a good stir and top with chopped nuts.

Serving Methods:

1. Layer with a dollop of Greek yogurt for added creaminess.

2. Sprinkle with additional pumpkin spice before serving.

Broccoli and Cheese Egg Muffins

Ingredients:

- 4 eggs

- 1 cup broccoli, finely chopped

- 1/2 cup cheddar cheese, shredded

- Salt and pepper to taste

Preparation Time: 10 minutes

Cooking Time: 15 minutes

Serving Time: 25 minutes

Nutritional Info:

- Calories: 220

- Protein: 15g

- Fiber: 3g

- Healthy Fats: 12g

Instructions:

- Preheat the oven to 350°F (175°C) and grease a muffin tin.

- Whisk eggs in a bowl, then add chopped broccoli, cheddar cheese, salt, and pepper.

- Pour the mixture into muffin cups and bake until eggs are set.

- Allow to cool slightly before serving.

Serving Methods:

1. Top with a dollop of Greek yogurt.

2. Serve with a side of whole-grain toast.

Mango and Coconut Chia Pudding

Ingredients:

- 3 tablespoons chia seeds

- 1 cup coconut milk

- 1 ripe mango, diced

- 1 tablespoon shredded coconut

Preparation Time: 5 minutes (plus overnight chilling)

Cooking Time: N/A

Serving Time: 10 minutes

Nutritional Info:

- Calories: 280

- Protein: 5g

- Fiber: 10g

- Healthy Fats: 15g

Instructions:

- Mix chia seeds and coconut milk in a bowl, refrigerate overnight.

- In the morning, layer chia pudding with diced mango in serving glasses.

- Top with shredded coconut.

Serving Methods:

1. Garnish with a drizzle of honey or agave syrup.

2. Sprinkle with chopped nuts for added crunch.

Turkey and Vegetable Breakfast Wrap

Ingredients:

- 1 whole-grain tortilla

- 2 scrambled eggs

- 2 slices turkey breast

- Spinach leaves

- Salsa for topping

Preparation Time: 10 minutes

Cooking Time: 5 minutes

Serving Time: 15 minutes

Nutritional Info:

- Calories: 300

- Protein: 20g

- Fiber: 4g

- Healthy Fats: 10g

Instructions:

- Scramble eggs and layer on a tortilla.

- Add turkey slices and spinach leaves.

- Roll into a wrap and top with salsa.

Serving Methods:

1. Serve with a side of fresh fruit.

2. Drizzle with a yogurt-based dressing.

Blueberry Almond Oat Bars

Ingredients:

- 1 cup rolled oats

- 1/2 cup almond butter

- 1/4 cup honey

- 1/2 cup blueberries

- 1/4 cup almond slices

Preparation Time: 15 minutes

Cooking Time: 20 minutes

Serving Time: 35 minutes

Nutritional Info:

- Calories: 250

- Protein: 7g

- Fiber: 5g

- Healthy Fats: 12g

Instructions:

- Preheat oven to 350°F (175°C) and line a baking dish with parchment paper.

- Mix rolled oats, almond butter, and honey in a bowl.

- Press half the mixture into the dish, add blueberries, and top with the remaining oat mixture.

- Sprinkle almond slices on top and bake until golden.

Serving Methods:

1. Cut into squares and serve with a dollop of yogurt.

2. Warm slightly and top with a scoop of vanilla ice cream.

Tomato Basil Mozzarella Omelette

Ingredients:

- 3 eggs

- 1/2 cup cherry tomatoes, halved

- Fresh basil leaves

- 1/4 cup mozzarella cheese, shredded

- Salt and pepper to taste

Preparation Time: 10 minutes

Cooking Time: 5 minutes

Serving Time: 15 minutes

Nutritional Info:

- Calories: 280

- Protein: 15g

- Fiber: 2g

- Healthy Fats: 18g

Instructions:

- Whisk eggs and season with salt and pepper.

- Pour into a heated skillet, add tomatoes, basil, and mozzarella.

- Fold into an omelette and cook until the cheese melts.

Serving Methods:

1. Garnish with a balsamic glaze.

2. Serve with a side of whole-grain toast.

Peach and Walnut Breakfast Quinoa

Ingredients:

- 1/2 cup cooked quinoa

- 1 peach, sliced

- 2 tablespoons walnuts, chopped

- 1 tablespoon honey

- Cinnamon for sprinkling

Preparation Time: 15 minutes

Cooking Time: 15 minutes (for quinoa)

Serving Time: 30 minutes

Nutritional Info:

- Calories: 290

- Protein: 7g

- Fiber: 5g

- Healthy Fats: 9g

Instructions:

- Combine cooked quinoa, peach slices, and walnuts in a bowl.

- Drizzle with honey and sprinkle with cinnamon.

- Mix well and serve.

Serving Methods:

1. Top with a dollop of Greek yogurt.

2. Garnish with mint leaves for freshness.

Pumpkin Pancakes with Maple Syrup

Ingredients:

- 1 cup pumpkin puree

- 1 cup whole wheat flour

- 1 teaspoon baking powder

- 1/2 teaspoon pumpkin spice

- Maple syrup for topping

Preparation Time: 10 minutes

Cooking Time: 10 minutes

Serving Time: 20 minutes

Nutritional Info:

- Calories: 220

- Protein: 6g

- Fiber: 4g

- Healthy Fats: 2g

Instructions:

- Mix pumpkin puree, whole wheat flour, baking powder, and pumpkin spice in a bowl.

- Heat a griddle, pour batter, and cook until bubbles appear.

- Flip and cook until both sides are golden.

Serving Methods:

1. Top with a scoop of vanilla yogurt.

2. Sprinkle with chopped pecans.

Smoked Salmon and Avocado Bagel

Ingredients:

- 1 whole-grain bagel

- 2 tablespoons cream cheese

- 2 ounces smoked salmon

- 1/2 avocado, sliced

- Capers and dill for garnish

Preparation Time: 10 minutes

Cooking Time: N/A

Serving Time: 15 minutes

Nutritional Info:

- Calories: 320

- Protein: 15g

- Fiber: 5g

- Healthy Fats: 15g

Instructions:

- Toast the bagel and spread cream cheese on each half.

- Layer with smoked salmon and sliced avocado.

- Garnish with capers and dill.

Serving Methods:

1. Squeeze fresh lemon juice on top.

2. Serve with a side of mixed greens.

Coconut Banana Baked Oatmeal

Ingredients:

- 1 cup rolled oats

- 1/2 cup shredded coconut

- 1 ripe banana, mashed

- 1 cup coconut milk

- 1 tablespoon maple syrup

Preparation Time: 10 minutes

Cooking Time: 25 minutes

Serving Time: 35 minutes

Nutritional Info:

- Calories: 270

- Protein: 5g

- Fiber: 6g

- Healthy Fats: 10g

Instructions:

- Preheat oven to 350°F (175°C) and grease a baking dish.

- Mix rolled oats, shredded coconut, mashed banana, coconut milk, and maple syrup.

- Pour into the baking dish and bake until set.

Serving Methods:

1. Top with a scoop of coconut or vanilla ice cream.

2. Drizzle with chocolate sauce for a treat.

Spinach and Mushroom Breakfast Quesadilla

Ingredients:

- 1 whole-grain tortilla

- 2 eggs, scrambled

- 1/2 cup spinach, chopped

- 1/4 cup mushrooms, sliced

- 1/4 cup cheddar cheese, shredded

Preparation Time: 10 minutes

Cooking Time: 10 minutes

Serving Time: 20 minutes

Nutritional Info:

- Calories: 280

- Protein: 15g

- Fiber: 4g

- Healthy Fats: 12g

Instructions:

- In a skillet, sauté spinach and mushrooms until wilted.

- Remove from the pan and scramble eggs.

- Lay the tortilla in the skillet, add eggs, sautéed vegetables, and cheddar cheese.

- Fold the tortilla and cook until cheese melts.

Serving Methods:

1. Serve with a side of salsa and guacamole.

2. Cut into wedges and enjoy with a dollop of sour cream.

CHAPTER FOUR

LUNCH RECIPES

Salmon and Quinoa Salad

Ingredients:

- 4 ounces grilled salmon

- 1/2 cup cooked quinoa

- Mixed greens

- Cherry tomatoes, halved

- Cucumber slices

- Olive oil and lemon dressing

Preparation Time: 15 minutes

Cooking Time: 15 minutes (for quinoa)

Serving Time: 30 minutes

Nutritional Info:

- Calories: 350

- Protein: 25g

- Fiber: 5g

- Healthy Fats: 15g

Instructions:

- Grill salmon and cook quinoa according to package instructions.

- In a bowl, combine quinoa, mixed greens, cherry tomatoes, and cucumber slices.

- Top with grilled salmon and drizzle with olive oil and lemon dressing.

Serving Methods:

1. Sprinkle with feta cheese or goat cheese.

2. Serve with a side of whole-grain bread.

Vegetarian Lentil Soup

Ingredients:

- 1 cup dried green lentils

- 1 onion, chopped

- 2 carrots, diced

- 2 celery stalks, chopped

- 3 cloves garlic, minced

- Vegetable broth

- Ground cumin and coriander

- Fresh parsley for garnish

Preparation Time: 15 minutes

Cooking Time: 30 minutes

Serving Time: 45 minutes

Nutritional Info:

- Calories: 250

- Protein: 15g

- Fiber: 12g

- Healthy Fats: 3g

Instructions:

- Rinse lentils and set aside.

- In a pot, sauté onion, carrots, celery, and garlic until softened.

- Add lentils, vegetable broth, cumin, and coriander. Simmer until lentils are tender.

- Garnish with fresh parsley before serving.

Serving Methods:

1. Serve with a dollop of Greek yogurt.

2. Pair with a whole-grain roll.

Chicken and Vegetable Stir-Fry

Ingredients:

- 4 ounces cooked chicken breast, sliced

- Broccoli florets

- Bell peppers, sliced

- Snap peas

- Low-sodium soy sauce

- Ginger and garlic for flavor

- Brown rice

Preparation Time: 20 minutes

Cooking Time: 15 minutes

Serving Time: 35 minutes

Nutritional Info:

- Calories: 300

- Protein: 20g

- Fiber: 6g

- Healthy Fats: 5g

Instructions:

- Cook chicken breast and set aside.

- In a wok, stir-fry broccoli, bell peppers, and snap peas.

- Add sliced chicken, soy sauce, ginger, and garlic. Stir until well combined.

- Serve over cooked brown rice.

Serving Methods:

1. Garnish with sesame seeds.

2. Drizzle with teriyaki sauce for extra flavor.

Sweet Potato and Black Bean Buddha Bowl

Ingredients:

- 1 medium sweet potato, roasted

- 1/2 cup black beans, cooked

- Quinoa

- Avocado slices

- Spinach leaves

- Tahini dressing

Preparation Time: 15 minutes

Cooking Time: 30 minutes (including roasting)

Serving Time: 45 minutes

Nutritional Info:

- Calories: 320

- Protein: 12g

- Fiber: 10g

- Healthy Fats: 10g

Instructions:

- Roast sweet potato in the oven until tender.

- Assemble a bowl with quinoa, black beans, roasted sweet potato, avocado slices, and spinach leaves.

- Drizzle with tahini dressing before serving.

Serving Methods:

- Top with pomegranate seeds for a burst of sweetness.

- Add a sprinkle of nutritional yeast for a cheesy flavor.

Turkey and Cranberry Wrap

Ingredients:

- 4 ounces sliced turkey breast

- Whole-grain wrap

- Cranberry sauce

- Baby spinach leaves

- Cream cheese

- Sliced almonds

Preparation Time: 10 minutes

Cooking Time: N/A

Serving Time: 15 minutes

Nutritional Info:

- Calories: 280

- Protein: 20g

- Fiber: 5g

- Healthy Fats: 8g

Instructions:

- Spread cream cheese on a whole-grain wrap.

- Layer with turkey slices, cranberry sauce, baby spinach, and sliced almonds.

- Roll into a wrap and slice before serving.

Serving Methods:

1. Toast the wrap for a warm option.

2. Serve with a side of vegetable sticks and hummus.

Caprese Salad with Grilled Chicken

Ingredients:

- 4 ounces grilled chicken breast, sliced

- Tomato slices

- Fresh mozzarella, sliced

- Fresh basil leaves

- Balsamic glaze

- Olive oil

- Salt and pepper

Preparation Time: 15 minutes

Cooking Time: 15 minutes

Serving Time: 30 minutes

Nutritional Info:

- Calories: 320

- Protein: 25g

- Fiber: 3g

- Healthy Fats: 15g

Instructions:

- Grill chicken breast and slice.

- Arrange tomato slices, fresh mozzarella, and grilled chicken on a plate.

- Drizzle with balsamic glaze and olive oil.

- Season with salt and pepper and garnish with fresh basil leaves.

Serving Methods:

1. Serve with a side of whole-grain bread.

2. Add a handful of mixed greens for extra freshness.

Mushroom and Spinach Quiche

Ingredients:

- Whole-grain pie crust

- 4 eggs

- 1 cup mushrooms, sliced

- 2 cups fresh spinach

- Feta cheese, crumbled

- Milk or non-dairy alternative

Preparation Time: 20 minutes

Cooking Time: 40 minutes

Serving Time: 1 hour

Nutritional Info:

- Calories: 280

- Protein: 15g

- Fiber: 4g

- Healthy Fats: 12g

Instructions:

- Preheat the oven and bake the pie crust according to the package instructions.

- In a skillet, sauté mushrooms and spinach until wilted.

- Whisk eggs with milk and season with salt and pepper.

- Layer mushroom and spinach mixture in the pie crust, pour egg mixture over, and sprinkle with feta.

- Bake until the quiche is set.

Serving Methods:

1. Serve with a side salad for a light meal.

2. Cut into squares for easy serving.

8. Cauliflower and Chickpea Curry

Ingredients:

- 1 cup cauliflower florets

- 1/2 cup chickpeas, cooked

- Coconut milk

- Curry powder and turmeric

- Basmati rice

- Fresh cilantro for garnish

Preparation Time: 15 minutes

Cooking Time: 25 minutes

Serving Time: 40 minutes

Nutritional Info:

- Calories: 300

- Protein: 10g

- Fiber: 8g

- Healthy Fats: 10g

Instructions:

- In a pot, simmer cauliflower and chickpeas in coconut milk with curry powder and turmeric.

- Cook until cauliflower is tender.

- Serve over basmati rice and garnish with fresh cilantro.

Serving Methods:

1. Top with a dollop of Greek yogurt.

2. Sprinkle with chopped cashews for crunch.

Eggplant and Tomato Stuffed Bell Peppers

Ingredients:

- Bell peppers, halved

- Eggplant, diced

- Tomatoes, chopped

- Quinoa

- Feta cheese

- Italian seasoning

- Olive oil

Preparation Time: 20 minutes

Cooking Time: 30 minutes

Serving Time: 50 minutes

Nutritional Info:

- Calories: 260

- Protein: 8g

- Fiber: 7g

- Healthy Fats: 9g

Instructions:

- Preheat the oven and roast bell peppers until slightly tender.

- In a skillet, sauté diced eggplant until golden, then add chopped tomatoes and Italian seasoning.

- Mix in cooked quinoa and feta cheese.

- Stuff bell peppers with the mixture and bake until cheese is melted.

Serving Methods:

1. Drizzle with balsamic reduction before serving.

2. Garnish with fresh basil for a burst of flavor.

Shrimp and Avocado Salad

Ingredients:

- 6 ounces cooked shrimp

- Mixed salad greens

- Avocado, sliced

- Cherry tomatoes, halved

- Cucumber slices

- Lime vinaigrette

Preparation Time: 15 minutes

Cooking Time: 5 minutes

Serving Time: 20 minutes

Nutritional Info:

- Calories: 280

- Protein: 20g

- Fiber: 6g

- Healthy Fats: 15g

Instructions:

- Cook shrimp and set aside.

- Assemble a salad with mixed greens, avocado slices, cherry tomatoes, and cucumber.

- Top with cooked shrimp and drizzle with lime vinaigrette.

Serving Methods:

1. Sprinkle with a pinch of chili flakes for heat.

2. Serve with a side of whole-grain crackers.

Quinoa and Vegetable Stir-Fry

Ingredients:

- 1 cup cooked quinoa

- Mixed vegetables (broccoli, bell peppers, snap peas)

- Tofu cubes

- Low-sodium soy sauce

- Sesame oil

- Garlic and ginger for flavor

Preparation Time: 15 minutes

Cooking Time: 15 minutes

Serving Time: 30 minutes

Nutritional Info:

- Calories: 280

- Protein: 15g

- Fiber: 7g

- Healthy Fats: 10g

Instructions:

- In a wok, stir-fry tofu and mixed vegetables in sesame oil.

- Add cooked quinoa and drizzle with low-sodium soy sauce.

- Stir until well combined and serve.

Serving Methods:

1. Top with crushed peanuts for added crunch.

2. Serve over a bed of spinach or kale.

Mediterranean Chickpea Salad

Ingredients:

- 1 can chickpeas, drained and rinsed

- Cherry tomatoes, halved

- Cucumber, diced

- Kalamata olives, sliced

- Feta cheese, crumbled

- Olive oil and lemon dressing

- Fresh parsley for garnish

Preparation Time: 15 minutes

Cooking Time: N/A

Serving Time: 20 minutes

Nutritional Info:

- Calories: 300

- Protein: 12g

- Fiber: 8g

- Healthy Fats: 15g

Instructions:

- In a bowl, combine chickpeas, cherry tomatoes, cucumber, olives, and feta.

- Drizzle with olive oil and lemon dressing, toss gently, and garnish with fresh parsley.

Serving Methods:

1. Serve on a bed of mixed greens.

2. Pair with whole-grain pita bread.

Salmon and Asparagus Foil Packets

Ingredients:

- 4 ounces salmon fillet

- Asparagus spears

- Lemon slices

- Garlic and dill for flavor

- Olive oil

- Salt and pepper to taste

Preparation Time: 15 minutes

Cooking Time: 20 minutes

Serving Time: 35 minutes

Nutritional Info:

- Calories: 320

- Protein: 25g

- Fiber: 5g

- Healthy Fats: 18g

Instructions:

- Preheat the oven and lay out a piece of foil.

- Place salmon fillet on the foil, surround with asparagus spears, and add lemon slices.

- Drizzle with olive oil, sprinkle with minced garlic and dill, season with salt and pepper.

- Seal the foil into a packet and bake until salmon is cooked through.

Serving Methods:

1. Serve with a side of quinoa or brown rice.

2. Garnish with extra fresh dill before serving.

Vegetable and Turkey Wrap

Ingredients:

- Whole-grain wrap

- 4 ounces lean ground turkey, cooked

- Hummus

- Mixed salad greens

- Tomatoes, sliced

- Red onion, thinly sliced

Preparation Time: 15 minutes

Cooking Time: 10 minutes

Serving Time: 25 minutes

Nutritional Info:

- Calories: 280

- Protein: 20g

- Fiber: 6g

- Healthy Fats: 10g

Instructions:

- Spread hummus on a whole-grain wrap.

- Layer with cooked ground turkey, mixed salad greens, sliced tomatoes, and red onion.

- Roll into a wrap and slice before serving.

Serving Methods:

1. Warm the wrap for a toasty option.

2. Serve with a side of carrot sticks and tzatziki.

Lentil and Spinach Curry

Ingredients:

- 1 cup dried green lentils

- Spinach leaves

- Onion, diced

- Tomatoes, chopped

- Coconut milk

- Curry spices (turmeric, cumin, coriander)

- Basmati rice

Preparation Time: 15 minutes

Cooking Time: 30 minutes

Serving Time: 45 minutes

Nutritional Info:

- Calories: 300

- Protein: 15g

- Fiber: 10g

- Healthy Fats: 8g

Instructions:

1. Rinse lentils and set aside.

2. In a pot, sauté diced onion until softened, then add chopped tomatoes and curry spices.

3. Add lentils, coconut milk, and cook until lentils are tender.

4. Stir in spinach leaves until wilted and serve over basmati rice.

Serving Methods:

- Garnish with a dollop of Greek yogurt.

- Sprinkle with fresh cilantro before serving.

Shrimp and Vegetable Skewers

Ingredients:

- Shrimp, peeled and deveined

- Bell peppers, cut into chunks

- Zucchini, sliced

- Cherry tomatoes

- Olive oil and lemon marinade

- Italian seasoning

- Skewers

Preparation Time: 20 minutes

Cooking Time: 10 minutes

Serving Time: 30 minutes

Nutritional Info:

- Calories: 250

- Protein: 20g

- Fiber: 4g

- Healthy Fats: 12g

Instructions:

- Preheat the grill or oven.

- Thread shrimp, bell peppers, zucchini, and cherry tomatoes onto skewers.

- Mix olive oil, lemon marinade, and Italian seasoning.

- Brush skewers with the marinade and grill until shrimp are cooked.

Serving Methods:

1. Serve over a bed of quinoa or couscous.

2. Drizzle with balsamic reduction before serving.

Turkey and Vegetable Stir-Fried Brown Rice

Ingredients:

- 4 ounces ground turkey, cooked

- Brown rice, cooked

- Mixed vegetables (carrots, peas, corn)

- Soy sauce

- Sesame oil

- Scallions, sliced

Preparation Time: 15 minutes

Cooking Time: 15 minutes

Serving Time: 30 minutes

Nutritional Info:

- Calories: 280

- Protein: 18g

- Fiber: 6g

- Healthy Fats: 8g

Instructions:

- Cook ground turkey and set aside.

- In a wok, stir-fry mixed vegetables with sesame oil.

- Add cooked brown rice and cooked turkey to the wok.

- Drizzle with soy sauce, stir until well combined, and garnish with sliced scallions.

Serving Methods:

1. Top with a fried egg for extra protein.

2. Sprinkle with sesame seeds before serving.

Chickpea and Vegetable Stew

Ingredients:

- 1 can chickpeas, drained and rinsed

- Carrots, diced

- Celery, chopped

- Onion, minced

- Garlic, minced

- Vegetable broth

- Italian herbs (rosemary, thyme)

- Spinach leaves

Preparation Time: 20 minutes

Cooking Time: 30 minutes

Serving Time: 50 minutes

Nutritional Info:

- Calories: 260

- Protein: 10g

- Fiber: 8g

- Healthy Fats: 5g

Instructions:

- In a pot, sauté minced onion and garlic until fragrant.

- Add diced carrots, chopped celery, and vegetable broth.

- Stir in chickpeas and Italian herbs, simmer until vegetables are tender.

- Add spinach leaves and cook until wilted.

Serving Methods:

1. Serve with a side of whole-grain bread.

2. Garnish with a dollop of pesto before serving.

Turkey and Vegetable Brown Rice Bowl

Ingredients:

- 4 ounces ground turkey, cooked

- Brown rice, cooked

- Broccoli florets

- Bell peppers, sliced

- Teriyaki sauce

- Sesame seeds for garnish

Preparation Time: 15 minutes

Cooking Time: 15 minutes

Serving Time: 30 minutes

Nutritional Info:

- Calories: 290

- Protein: 20g

- Fiber: 7g

- Healthy Fats: 8g

Instructions:

- Cook ground turkey and set aside.

- In a skillet, sauté broccoli florets and sliced bell peppers.

- Add cooked brown rice and turkey to the skillet.

- Drizzle with teriyaki sauce, stir until heated through, and sprinkle with sesame seeds.

Serving Methods:

- Top with sliced green onions before serving.

- Serve in a bowl with chopsticks for an Asian-inspired experience.

Egg Salad Lettuce Wraps

Ingredients:

- Hard-boiled eggs, chopped

- Greek yogurt

- Mustard

- Celery, finely chopped

- Lettuce leaves

- Cherry tomatoes, halved

- Avocado slices

Preparation Time: 15 minutes

Cooking Time: N/A

Serving Time: 20 minutes

Nutritional Info:

- Calories: 240

- Protein: 15g

- Fiber: 5g

- Healthy Fats: 14g

Instructions:

- In a bowl, mix chopped hard-boiled eggs, Greek yogurt, mustard, and finely chopped celery.

- Spoon the egg salad into lettuce leaves.

- Garnish with cherry tomatoes and avocado slices.

Serving Methods:

1. Sprinkle with paprika for a pop of color.

2. Serve with a side of fresh fruit.

CHAPTER FIVE

DINNER RECIPES

Baked Lemon Herb Chicken

Ingredients:

- 4 boneless, skinless chicken breasts

- Lemon juice

- Garlic powder

- Dried thyme

- Olive oil

- Salt and pepper

Preparation Time: 15 minutes

Cooking Time: 25 minutes

Serving Time: 40 minutes

Nutritional Info:

- Calories: 280

- Protein: 30g

- Fiber: 2g

- Healthy Fats: 10g

Instructions:

- Preheat the oven to 400°F (200°C).

- Place chicken breasts in a baking dish.

- Drizzle with lemon juice, olive oil, and sprinkle with garlic powder, thyme, salt, and pepper.

- Bake until chicken is cooked through.

Serving Methods:

1. Serve with steamed broccoli and quinoa.

2. Pair with a side of roasted sweet potatoes.

Vegetarian Stuffed Bell Peppers

Ingredients:

- Bell peppers, halved

- Quinoa

- Black beans, drained and rinsed

- Corn kernels

- Salsa

- Cumin and chili powder

- Shredded cheese

Preparation Time: 20 minutes

Cooking Time: 30 minutes

Serving Time: 50 minutes

Nutritional Info:

- Calories: 320

- Protein: 15g

- Fiber: 8g

- Healthy Fats: 10g

Instructions:

- Preheat the oven to 375°F (190°C).

- Cook quinoa according to package instructions.

- In a bowl, mix cooked quinoa, black beans, corn, salsa, cumin, and chili powder.

- Spoon the mixture into halved bell peppers, top with shredded cheese, and bake until peppers are tender.

Serving Methods:

1. Drizzle with avocado crema before serving.

2. Garnish with fresh cilantro.

Salmon and Sweet Potato Foil Packets

Ingredients:

- 4 ounces' salmon fillet

- Sweet potato, thinly sliced

- Broccoli florets

- Lemon slices

- Dill and garlic for flavor

- Olive oil

- Salt and pepper

Preparation Time: 15 minutes

Cooking Time: 25 minutes

Serving Time: 40 minutes

Nutritional Info:

- Calories: 310

- Protein: 25g

- Fiber: 6g

- Healthy Fats: 15g

Instructions:

- Preheat the oven to 400°F (200°C).

- Lay out a piece of foil and place sweet potato slices.

- Top with salmon, broccoli, lemon slices, dill, garlic, olive oil, salt, and pepper.

- Seal into a packet and bake until salmon is cooked.

Serving Methods:

1. Serve with a side of quinoa or brown rice.

2. Top with a dollop of Greek yogurt.

Turkey and Vegetable Skillet

Ingredients:

- 4 ounces ground turkey

- Quinoa

- Bell peppers, diced

- Zucchini, sliced

- Tomato sauce

- Italian herbs (oregano, basil)

- Parmesan cheese

Preparation Time: 20 minutes

Cooking Time: 20 minutes

Serving Time: 40 minutes

Nutritional Info:

- Calories: 290
- Protein: 18g
- Fiber: 5g
- Healthy Fats: 8g

Instructions:

- Cook ground turkey in a skillet.
- Add diced bell peppers, sliced zucchini, tomato sauce, and Italian herbs.
- Simmer until vegetables are tender.
- Serve over cooked quinoa and sprinkle with Parmesan cheese.

Serving Methods:

1. Garnish with fresh basil before serving.
2. Serve with a side of mixed greens.

Cauliflower Fried Rice with Shrimp

Ingredients:

- Cauliflower rice
- Shrimp, peeled and deveined

- Mixed vegetables (peas, carrots, corn)

- Soy sauce

- Ginger and garlic

- Green onions, sliced

- Sesame oil

Preparation Time: 20 minutes

Cooking Time: 15 minutes

Serving Time: 35 minutes

Nutritional Info:

- Calories: 250

- Protein: 20g

- Fiber: 6g

- Healthy Fats: 10g

Instructions:

- In a wok, stir-fry shrimp until cooked.

- Add mixed vegetables, cauliflower rice, soy sauce, ginger, and garlic.

- Stir until well combined, and finish with a drizzle of sesame oil.

- Garnish with sliced green onions.

Serving Methods:

1. Serve with a side of edamame.

2. Top with a fried egg for extra protein.

Mushroom and Spinach Stuffed Chicken Breast

Ingredients:

- 2 boneless, skinless chicken breasts

- Mushrooms, chopped

- Spinach leaves

- Feta cheese

- Olive oil

- Garlic and thyme for flavor

- Salt and pepper

Preparation Time: 25 minutes

Cooking Time: 30 minutes

Serving Time: 55 minutes

Nutritional Info:

- Calories: 290

- Protein: 30g

- Fiber: 4g

- Healthy Fats: 12g

Instructions:

- Preheat the oven to 375°F (190°C).

- In a skillet, sauté chopped mushrooms with garlic and thyme.

- Butterfly chicken breasts and stuff with sautéed mushrooms, spinach, and feta.

- Secure with toothpicks, brush with olive oil, and bake until chicken is cooked through.

Serving Methods:

1. Serve with a side of roasted Brussels sprouts.

2. Drizzle with balsamic reduction before serving.

Vegetable and Lentil Curry

Ingredients:

- 1 cup dried green lentils

- Mixed vegetables (carrots, peas, cauliflower)

- Coconut milk

- Curry powder and turmeric

- Basmati rice

- Fresh cilantro for garnish

Preparation Time: 20 minutes

Cooking Time: 30 minutes

Serving Time: 50 minutes

Nutritional Info:

- Calories: 280

- Protein: 15g

- Fiber: 8g

- Healthy Fats: 10g

Instructions:

- Rinse lentils and set aside.

- In a pot, simmer lentils, mixed vegetables, coconut milk, curry powder, and turmeric.

- Cook until lentils are tender.

- Serve over basmati rice and garnish with fresh cilantro.

Serving Methods:

1. Top with a dollop of Greek yogurt.

2. Sprinkle with chopped cashews for crunch.

Pesto Zoodles with Grilled Chicken

Ingredients:

- Zucchini noodles (zoodles)

- 4 ounces grilled chicken breast

- Cherry tomatoes, halved

- Pesto sauce

- Pine nuts for garnish

- Parmesan cheese

Preparation Time: 15 minutes

Cooking Time: 15 minutes

Serving Time: 30 minutes

Nutritional Info:

- Calories: 320

- Protein: 25g

- Fiber: 5g

- Healthy Fats: 15g

Instructions:

- Spiralize zucchini into noodles.

- Grill chicken breast and slice.

- In a pan, sauté zoodles with cherry tomatoes and pesto sauce until heated through.

- Top with grilled chicken, pine nuts, and Parmesan cheese.

Serving Methods:

1. Sprinkle with red pepper flakes for a kick.

2. Serve with a side of garlic bread.

Baked Cod with Lemon Dill Sauce

Ingredients:

- Cod fillets

- Lemon zest and juice

- Fresh dill, chopped

- Garlic powder

- Olive oil

- Salt and pepper

Preparation Time: 15 minutes

Cooking Time: 20 minutes

Serving Time: 35 minutes

Nutritional Info:

- Calories: 260

- Protein: 30g

- Fiber: 1g

- Healthy Fats: 12g

Instructions:

- Preheat the oven to 400°F (200°C).

- Place cod fillets in a baking dish.

- Mix lemon zest, lemon juice, chopped dill, garlic powder, olive oil, salt, and pepper.

- Drizzle the mixture over the cod and bake until fish is flaky.

Serving Methods:

1. Serve with a side of quinoa and steamed green beans.

2. Garnish with extra fresh dill before serving.

Chickpea and Vegetable Stir-Fry

Ingredients:

- 1 can chickpeas, drained and rinsed

- Mixed vegetables (bell peppers, snap peas, carrots)

- Brown rice

- Soy sauce

- Ginger and garlic for flavor

- Sesame oil

- Green onions, sliced

Preparation Time: 20 minutes

Cooking Time: 15 minutes

Serving Time: 35 minutes

Nutritional Info:

- Calories: 300

- Protein: 12g

- Fiber: 8g

- Healthy Fats: 10g

Instructions:

- In a wok, stir-fry mixed vegetables and chickpeas in sesame oil.

- Add soy sauce, ginger, and garlic. Stir until well combined.

- Serve over cooked brown rice and garnish with sliced green onions.

Serving Methods:

1. Top with crushed peanuts for added texture.

2. Pair with a side of vegetable spring rolls.

1. Grilled Turkey and Vegetable Kebabs

Ingredients:

- 4 ounces' turkey breast, cut into chunks

- Bell peppers, cherry tomatoes, and zucchini, cut into chunks

- Olive oil and lemon marinade

- Rosemary and garlic for flavor

- Salt and pepper

Preparation Time: 20 minutes

Cooking Time: 15 minutes

Serving Time: 35 minutes

Nutritional Info:

- Calories: 280

- Protein: 20g

- Fiber: 6g

- Healthy Fats: 10g

Instructions:

- In a bowl, marinate turkey chunks in olive oil, lemon, rosemary, garlic, salt, and pepper.

- Thread turkey and vegetables onto skewers.

- Grill until turkey is cooked and vegetables are tender.

Serving Methods:

1. Serve over a bed of quinoa.

2. Drizzle with balsamic glaze before serving.

Eggplant Parmesan

Ingredients:

- Eggplant slices

- Marinara sauce

- Mozzarella and Parmesan cheese

- Whole-wheat breadcrumbs

- Egg

- Basil and oregano for flavor

- Olive oil

Preparation Time: 25 minutes

Cooking Time: 30 minutes

Serving Time: 55 minutes

Nutritional Info:

- Calories: 320

- Protein: 15g

- Fiber: 8g

- Healthy Fats: 12g

Instructions:

- Preheat the oven to 375°F (190°C).

- Dip eggplant slices in beaten egg and coat with whole-wheat breadcrumbs.

- Bake until golden brown.

- Layer baked eggplant with marinara sauce and cheeses, then bake until cheese is melted.

Serving Methods:

1. Serve with a side of whole-grain pasta.

2. Garnish with fresh basil before serving.

Salmon and Spinach Stuffed Portobello Mushrooms

Ingredients:

- Portobello mushrooms, stems removed

- 4 ounces' salmon fillet, cooked and flaked

- Fresh spinach leaves

- Feta cheese

- Lemon zest

- Olive oil

- Garlic powder

Preparation Time: 20 minutes

Cooking Time: 20 minutes

Serving Time: 40 minutes

Nutritional Info:

- Calories: 300

- Protein: 25g

- Fiber: 4g

- Healthy Fats: 15g

Instructions:

- Preheat the oven to 375°F (190°C).

- Brush Portobello mushrooms with olive oil and sprinkle with garlic powder.

- Layer mushrooms with fresh spinach, cooked salmon, and feta cheese.

- Bake until mushrooms are tender.

Serving Methods:

1. Serve with a side of quinoa or wild rice.

2. Drizzle with a balsamic reduction before serving.

Vegetarian Chickpea and Sweet Potato Curry

Ingredients:

- 1 can chickpeas, drained and rinsed

- Sweet potatoes, diced

- Coconut milk

- Curry powder and turmeric

- Onion and garlic, minced

- Basmati rice

Preparation Time: 20 minutes

Cooking Time: 30 minutes

Serving Time: 50 minutes

Nutritional Info:

- Calories: 280

- Protein: 12g

- Fiber: 8g

- Healthy Fats: 10g

Instructions:

- In a pot, sauté minced onion and garlic until fragrant.

- Add diced sweet potatoes, chickpeas, coconut milk, curry powder, and turmeric.

- Simmer until sweet potatoes are tender.

- Serve over basmati rice.

Serving Methods:

1. Garnish with fresh cilantro before serving.

2. Top with a dollop of Greek yogurt.

Teriyaki Chicken Stir-Fry

Ingredients:

- 4 ounces' chicken breast, sliced

- Broccoli florets

- Carrots, julienned

- Snap peas

- Brown rice

- Teriyaki sauce

- Sesame oil

- Green onions, sliced

Preparation Time: 20 minutes

Cooking Time: 15 minutes

Serving Time: 35 minutes

Nutritional Info:

- Calories: 320

- Protein: 25g

- Fiber: 6g

- Healthy Fats: 10g

Instructions:

- Cook sliced chicken in a wok with sesame oil until browned.

- Add broccoli, carrots, and snap peas. Stir-fry until vegetables are tender-crisp.

- Drizzle with teriyaki sauce and stir until well coated.

- Serve over cooked brown rice and garnish with sliced green onions.

Serving Methods:

1. Top with crushed cashews before serving.

2. Sprinkle with sesame seeds for added texture.

Quinoa and Black Bean Stuffed Peppers

Ingredients:

- Bell peppers, halved

- 1 cup cooked quinoa

- Black beans, drained and rinsed

- Corn kernels

- Salsa

- Cumin and chili powder

- Shredded cheese

Preparation Time: 25 minutes

Cooking Time: 30 minutes

Serving Time: 55 minutes

Nutritional Info:

- Calories: 310

- Protein: 15g

- Fiber: 8g

- Healthy Fats: 12g

Instructions:

- Preheat the oven to 375°F (190°C).

- In a bowl, mix cooked quinoa, black beans, corn, salsa, cumin, and chili powder.

- Spoon the mixture into halved bell peppers and top with shredded cheese.

- Bake until peppers are tender and cheese is melted.

Serving Methods:

1. Garnish with avocado slices before serving.

2. Serve with a side of guacamole.

Lemon Garlic Shrimp and Broccoli Pasta

Ingredients:

- 6 ounces whole-grain pasta

- 6 ounces' shrimp, peeled and deveined

- Broccoli florets

- Lemon zest and juice

- Garlic, minced

- Olive oil

- Red pepper flakes

Preparation Time: 20 minutes

Cooking Time: 15 minutes

Serving Time: 35 minutes

Nutritional Info:

- Calories: 340

- Protein: 20g

- Fiber: 7g

- Healthy Fats: 12g

Instructions:

- Cook pasta according to package instructions.

- In a skillet, cook shrimp in olive oil with minced garlic.

- Add broccoli, lemon zest, and juice. Cook until broccoli is tender.

- Toss with cooked pasta and sprinkle with red pepper flakes.

Serving Methods:

1. Garnish with chopped parsley before serving.

2. Serve with a side of mixed greens.

Baked Herb-Crusted Cod

Ingredients:

- Cod fillets

- Whole-grain breadcrumbs

- Fresh herbs (parsley, thyme)

- Lemon zest

- Dijon mustard

- Olive oil

- Salt and pepper

Preparation Time: 15 minutes

Cooking Time: 20 minutes

Serving Time: 35 minutes

Nutritional Info:

- Calories: 290

- Protein: 30g

- Fiber: 2g

- Healthy Fats: 15g

Instructions:

- Preheat the oven to 400°F (200°C).

- Mix whole-grain breadcrumbs with chopped herbs, lemon zest, Dijon mustard, olive oil, salt, and pepper.

- Coat cod fillets with the mixture and bake until fish is flaky.

Serving Methods:

1. Serve with a side of quinoa and steamed asparagus.

2. Drizzle with a lemon-dill sauce before serving.

Vegetable and Chickpea Stir-Fry

Ingredients:

- 1 can chickpeas, drained and rinsed

- Mixed vegetables (bell peppers, broccoli, snow peas)

- Brown rice

- Soy sauce

- Ginger and garlic for flavor

- Sesame oil

- Cashews for garnish

Preparation Time: 20 minutes

Cooking Time: 15 minutes

Serving Time: 35 minutes

Nutritional Info:

- Calories: 310

- Protein: 14g

- Fiber: 7g

- Healthy Fats: 10g

Instructions:

- In a wok, stir-fry mixed vegetables and chickpeas in sesame oil.

- Add soy sauce, ginger, and garlic. Stir until well combined.

- Serve over cooked brown rice and garnish with cashews.

Serving Methods:

1. Top with sliced green onions before serving.

2. Pair with a side of vegetable spring rolls.

Mango Glazed Chicken Skewers

Ingredients:

- 4 ounces' chicken breast, cut into chunks

- Mango, pureed

- Lime juice

- Honey

- Chili powder

- Cilantro, chopped

- Salt and pepper

Preparation Time: 20 minutes

Cooking Time: 15 minutes

Serving Time: 35 minutes

Nutritional Info:

- Calories: 270

- Protein: 18g

- Fiber: 3g

- Healthy Fats: 8g

Instructions:

- In a bowl, mix mango puree, lime juice, honey, chili powder, cilantro, salt, and pepper.

- Marinate chicken chunks in the mixture.

- Thread chicken onto skewers and grill until cooked through.

Serving Methods:

1. Serve over a bed of coconut rice.

2. Drizzle with extra mango glaze before serving.

CHAPTER SIX

SNACKS AND APPETIZERS

Chia Seed Pudding Parfait

Ingredients:

- 2 tablespoons chia seeds

- 1 cup almond milk

- Greek yogurt

- Mixed berries (blueberries, raspberries)

- Honey

- Granola

Preparation Time: 10 minutes (plus overnight chilling)

Cooking Time: N/A

Serving Time: 15 minutes

Nutritional Info:

- Calories: 180

- Protein: 6g

- Fiber: 8g

- Healthy Fats: 5g

Instructions:

- Mix chia seeds and almond milk, refrigerate overnight.

- In a glass, layer chia pudding with Greek yogurt, mixed berries, and granola.

- Drizzle with honey.

Serving Methods:

- Top with a sprinkle of cinnamon before serving.

- Serve as a refreshing breakfast or afternoon snack.

Sweet Potato and Rosemary Bites

Ingredients:

- Sweet potatoes, thinly sliced

- Olive oil

- Fresh rosemary, chopped

- Sea salt

- Greek yogurt dip (optional)

Preparation Time: 15 minutes

Cooking Time: 20 minutes

Serving Time: 35 minutes

Nutritional Info:

- Calories: 100

- Protein: 2g

- Fiber: 3g

- Healthy Fats: 4g

Instructions:

- Preheat the oven to 400°F (200°C).

- Toss sweet potato slices in olive oil, rosemary, and sea salt.

- Bake until crispy.

- Serve with a side of Greek yogurt dip.

Serving Methods:

- Sprinkle with a touch of paprika before serving.

- Arrange on a platter for a party appetizer.

Cottage Cheese Stuffed Strawberries

Ingredients:

- Fresh strawberries, hulled

- Cottage cheese

- Almonds, chopped

- Honey

Preparation Time: 10 minutes

Cooking Time: N/A

Serving Time: 15 minutes

Nutritional Info:

- Calories: 80

- Protein: 5g

- Fiber: 2g

- Healthy Fats: 4g

Instructions:

- Fill each strawberry with cottage cheese.

- Top with chopped almonds and drizzle with honey.

Serving Methods:

1. Sprinkle with a pinch of cinnamon before serving.

2. Arrange on a dessert platter.

Mango Salsa with Cucumber Chips

Ingredients:

- Mango, diced

- Red onion, finely chopped

- Jalapeño, minced

- Cilantro, chopped

- Lime juice

- Cucumber, sliced

Preparation Time: 15 minutes

Cooking Time: N/A

Serving Time: 20 minutes

Nutritional Info:

- Calories: 70

- Protein: 1g

- Fiber: 2g

- Healthy Fats: 0g

Instructions:

- Mix mango, red onion, jalapeño, cilantro, and lime juice.

- Use cucumber slices as chips for dipping.

Serving Methods:

1. Top with crumbled feta for added flavor.

2. Serve in individual bowls for easy snacking.

Edamame and Mint Hummus

Ingredients:

- 1 cup edamame, shelled

- Chickpeas, drained and rinsed

- Mint leaves

- Tahini

- Lemon juice

- Garlic, minced

- Pita bread triangles

Preparation Time: 20 minutes

Cooking Time: 5 minutes

Serving Time: 25 minutes

Nutritional Info:

- Calories: 120

- Protein: 7g

- Fiber: 4g

- Healthy Fats: 5g

Instructions:

- Boil edamame until tender.

- Blend edamame, chickpeas, mint, tahini, lemon juice, and garlic until smooth.

- Serve with pita bread triangles.

Serving Methods:

1. Garnish with a drizzle of olive oil before serving.

2. Use as a spread for vegetable wraps.

Tomato Basil Bruschetta

Ingredients:

- Tomatoes, diced

- Fresh basil, chopped

- Garlic, minced

- Balsamic vinegar

- Olive oil

- Whole-grain baguette slices

Preparation Time: 15 minutes

Cooking Time: 5 minutes

Serving Time: 20 minutes

Nutritional Info:

- Calories: 90

- Protein: 3g

- Fiber: 2g

- Healthy Fats: 4g

Instructions:

- In a bowl, mix tomatoes, basil, garlic, balsamic vinegar, and olive oil.

- Toast whole-grain baguette slices and top with the tomato mixture.

Serving Methods:

1. Sprinkle with a pinch of sea salt before serving.

2. Serve as an appetizer for a light meal.

Almond Butter and Banana Bites

Ingredients:

- Whole-grain crackers

- Almond butter

- Banana slices

- Chia seeds (optional)

Preparation Time: 10 minutes

Cooking Time: N/A

Serving Time: 15 minutes

Nutritional Info:

- Calories: 120

- Protein: 3g

- Fiber: 3g

- Healthy Fats: 6g

Instructions:

- Spread almond butter on whole-grain crackers.

- Top with banana slices and sprinkle with chia seeds.

Serving Methods:

1. Drizzle with honey for a touch of sweetness.

2. Serve on a wooden board for a charming presentation.

Pumpkin Seeds and Cranberry Mix

Ingredients:

- Pumpkin seeds (pepitas)

- Dried cranberries

- Dark chocolate chips

- Cinnamon

Preparation Time: 10 minutes

Cooking Time: N/A

Serving Time: 15 minutes

Nutritional Info:

- Calories: 110

- Protein: 4g

- Fiber: 2g

- Healthy Fats: 5g

Instructions:

- Mix pumpkin seeds, dried cranberries, and dark chocolate chips.

- Sprinkle with cinnamon for flavor.

Serving Methods:

1. Serve in small jars for portion control.

2. Mix into Greek yogurt for a crunchy parfait.

Caprese Skewers

Ingredients:

- Cherry tomatoes

- Mozzarella balls

- Fresh basil leaves

- Balsamic glaze

Preparation Time: 15 minutes

Cooking Time: N/A

Serving Time: 20 minutes

Nutritional Info:

- Calories: 100

- Protein: 5g

- Fiber: 1g

- Healthy Fats: 7g

Instructions:

- Thread cherry tomatoes, mozzarella balls, and fresh basil leaves onto skewers.

- Drizzle with balsamic glaze.

Serving Methods:

1. Sprinkle with a pinch of sea salt before serving.

2. Serve on a platter for a stylish appetizer.

Guacamole-Stuffed Cucumber Cups

Ingredients:

- Cucumbers, sliced into rounds

- Avocados, mashed

- Tomatoes, diced

- Red onion, finely chopped

- Lime juice

- Cilantro, chopped

Preparation Time: 15 minutes

Cooking Time: N/A

Serving Time: 20 minutes

Nutritional Info:

- Calories: 90

- Protein: 2g

- Fiber: 3g

- Healthy Fats: 7g

Instructions:

- Scoop out a small portion from each cucumber round to create a cup.

- In a bowl, mix mashed avocados, diced tomatoes, red onion, lime juice, and cilantro.

- Fill each cucumber cup with guacamole.

Serving Methods:

1. Garnish with a sprinkle of chili powder before serving.

2. Serve on a colorful platter for a festive display.

Quinoa and Vegetable Stuffed Bell Peppers

Ingredients:

- Bell peppers, halved

- Quinoa, cooked

- Mixed vegetables (zucchini, carrots, peas)

- Olive oil

- Garlic powder

- Fresh herbs (parsley, thyme)

- Salt and pepper

Preparation Time: 20 minutes

Cooking Time: 30 minutes

Serving Time: 50 minutes

Nutritional Info:

- Calories: 120

- Protein: 5g

- Fiber: 4g

- Healthy Fats: 3g

Instructions:

- Preheat the oven to 375°F (190°C).

- In a skillet, sauté mixed vegetables in olive oil until tender.

- Mix cooked quinoa with sautéed vegetables, garlic powder, fresh herbs, salt, and pepper.

- Stuff bell peppers with the quinoa and vegetable mixture and bake until peppers are tender.

Serving Methods:

1. Drizzle with a balsamic reduction before serving.

2. Serve as an appetizer or side dish.

Smoked Salmon Cucumber Bites

Ingredients:

- English cucumber, sliced

- Smoked salmon

- Cream cheese

- Capers

- Dill, for garnish

- Lemon zest

Preparation Time: 15 minutes

Cooking Time: N/A

Serving Time: 20 minutes

Nutritional Info:

- Calories: 80

- Protein: 5g

- Fiber: 1g

- Healthy Fats: 4g

Instructions:

- Lay cucumber slices on a serving platter.

- Top each slice with a small amount of cream cheese, a piece of smoked salmon, and a few capers.

- Garnish with fresh dill and lemon zest.

Serving Methods:

1. Sprinkle with black pepper before serving.

2. Serve as an elegant appetizer for gatherings.

Roasted Chickpeas

Ingredients:

- 1 can chickpeas, drained and rinsed

- Olive oil

- Smoked paprika

- Cumin

- Garlic powder

- Salt

Preparation Time: 10 minutes

Cooking Time: 30 minutes

Serving Time: 40 minutes

Nutritional Info:

- Calories: 90

- Protein: 4g

- Fiber: 4g

- Healthy Fats: 3g

Instructions:

- Preheat the oven to 400°F (200°C).

- Toss chickpeas with olive oil, smoked paprika, cumin, garlic powder, and salt.

- Roast in the oven until crispy.

Serving Methods:

1. Sprinkle with nutritional yeast for a cheesy flavor.

2. Serve in small bowls for a crunchy snack.

Zucchini and Goat Cheese Roll-Ups

Ingredients:

- Zucchini, thinly sliced

- Goat cheese

- Sun-dried tomatoes, chopped

- Basil leaves

- Balsamic glaze

Preparation Time: 15 minutes

Cooking Time: N/A

Serving Time: 20 minutes

Nutritional Info:

- Calories: 100

- Protein: 5g

- Fiber: 2g

- Healthy Fats: 4g

Instructions:

1. Lay zucchini slices flat.

2. Spread a thin layer of goat cheese on each slice.

3. Top with sun-dried tomatoes and a basil leaf.

4. Roll up each slice and secure with a toothpick.

5. Drizzle with balsamic glaze before serving.

Serving Methods:

- Garnish with pine nuts for added texture.

- Serve as a light and flavorful appetizer.

Mushroom and Spinach Stuffed Phyllo Cups

Ingredients:

- Phyllo dough cups

- Mushrooms, chopped

- Spinach, chopped

- Feta cheese, crumbled

- Onion, finely chopped

- Olive oil

- Black pepper

Preparation Time: 20 minutes

Cooking Time: 15 minutes

Serving Time: 35 minutes

Nutritional Info:

- Calories: 110

- Protein: 4g

- Fiber: 1g

- Healthy Fats: 5g

Instructions:

- Preheat the oven to 350°F (175°C).

- In a skillet, sauté mushrooms, spinach, and onion in olive oil until cooked.

- Fill phyllo dough cups with the sautéed mixture and top with crumbled feta.

- Bake until phyllo is golden brown.

Serving Methods:

1. Garnish with a sprinkle of nutmeg before serving.

2. Serve as bite-sized appetizers for parties.

Tuna Salad Lettuce Wraps

Ingredients:

- Canned tuna, drained

- Greek yogurt

- Celery, finely chopped

- Red onion, finely chopped

- Dill, chopped

- Lettuce leaves (such as Bibb or Romaine)

Preparation Time: 15 minutes

Cooking Time: N/A

Serving Time: 20 minutes

Nutritional Info:

- Calories: 90

- Protein: 12g

- Fiber: 1g

- Healthy Fats: 2g

Instructions:

- In a bowl, mix canned tuna, Greek yogurt, celery, red onion, and chopped dill.

- Spoon the tuna salad onto individual lettuce leaves.

- Roll up the leaves to create wraps.

Serving Methods:

1. Sprinkle with lemon juice before serving.

2. Serve as a light lunch or appetizer.

Cauliflower Buffalo Bites

Ingredients:

- Cauliflower florets

- Buffalo sauce

- Whole-wheat flour

- Garlic powder

- Onion powder

- Greek yogurt ranch dip

Preparation Time: 15 minutes

Cooking Time: 25 minutes

Serving Time: 40 minutes

Nutritional Info:

- Calories: 80
- Protein: 3g
- Fiber: 2g
- Healthy Fats: 2g

Instructions:

- Preheat the oven to 425°F (220°C).
- In a bowl, toss cauliflower florets with whole-wheat flour, garlic powder, and onion powder.
- Bake until crispy and toss in buffalo sauce.
- Serve with Greek yogurt ranch dip.

Serving Methods:

1. Garnish with chopped chives before serving.
2. Serve as a healthier alternative to buffalo wings.

Egg Salad Stuffed Cucumber Cups

Ingredients:

- Cucumbers, sliced into rounds
- Hard-boiled eggs, chopped
- Greek yogurt

- Dijon mustard

- Chives, chopped

- Paprika

Preparation Time: 15 minutes

Cooking Time: N/A

Serving Time: 20 minutes

Nutritional Info:

- Calories: 70

- Protein: 5g

- Fiber: 1g

- Healthy Fats: 4g

Instructions:

- Scoop out a small portion from each cucumber round to create a cup.

- In a bowl, mix chopped hard-boiled eggs, Greek yogurt, Dijon mustard, and chives.

- Fill each cucumber cup with the egg salad and sprinkle with paprika.

Serving Methods:

1. Garnish with a slice of cherry tomato before serving.

2. Serve as a refreshing snack or appetizer.

Sesame Ginger Snap Peas

Ingredients:

- Snap peas, trimmed

- Sesame oil

- Soy sauce

- Fresh ginger, grated

- Sesame seeds

- Green onions, sliced

Preparation Time: 10 minutes

Cooking Time: 5 minutes

Serving Time: 15 minutes

Nutritional Info:

- Calories: 60

- Protein: 2g

- Fiber: 2g

- Healthy Fats: 3g

Instructions:

- In a wok, stir-fry snap peas in sesame oil until slightly tender.

- Add soy sauce, grated fresh ginger, and sesame seeds.

- Toss until well coated.

Serving Methods:

1. Squeeze fresh lime juice before serving.

2. Serve as a crunchy and flavorful snack.

Peach and Goat Cheese Crostini

Ingredients:

- Whole-grain baguette, sliced

- Goat cheese

- Fresh peaches, sliced

- Honey

- Thyme leaves for garnish

Preparation Time: 15 minutes

Cooking Time: 5 minutes

Serving Time: 20 minutes

Nutritional Info:

- Calories: 100

- Protein: 4g

- Fiber: 2g

- Healthy Fats: 3g

Instructions:

- Toast whole-grain baguette slices.

- Spread a layer of goat cheese on each slice.

- Top with fresh peach slices and drizzle with honey.

- Garnish with thyme leaves.

Serving Methods:

1. Sprinkle with crushed pistachios before serving.

2. Serve as a sweet and savory appetizer

CHAPTER SEVEN

DESSERTS WITH BENEFITS

Berry Yogurt Parfait

Ingredients:

- Greek yogurt

- Mixed berries (blueberries, strawberries)

- Walnuts, chopped

- Honey

Preparation Time: 10 minutes

Cooking Time: N/A

Serving Time: 15 minutes

Nutritional Info:

- Calories: 150

- Protein: 8g

- Fiber: 4g

- Healthy Fats: 6g

Benefits:

- Rich in antioxidants from berries.

- Provides Omega-3 fatty acids from walnuts.

Instructions:

- In a glass, layer Greek yogurt with mixed berries and chopped walnuts.

- Drizzle with honey.

- Repeat layers and serve chilled.

Serving Methods:

1. Top with a sprinkle of chia seeds for added texture.

2. Serve as a light and refreshing dessert after meals.

Avocado Chocolate Mousse

Ingredients:

- Ripe avocados

- Cocoa powder

- Maple syrup

- Vanilla extract

- Almond milk

Preparation Time: 15 minutes

Cooking Time: N/A

Serving Time: 30 minutes

Nutritional Info:

- Calories: 180

- Protein: 3g

- Fiber: 6g

- Healthy Fats: 12g

Benefits:

- Avocados provide healthy monounsaturated fats.

- Cocoa powder is rich in antioxidants.

Instructions:

- Blend avocados, cocoa powder, maple syrup, vanilla extract, and almond milk until smooth.

- Chill in the refrigerator.

- Serve in small bowls.

Serving Methods:

1. Garnish with a dollop of whipped coconut cream.

2. Serve as a guilt-free chocolate indulgence.

Chia Seed and Mango Pudding

Ingredients:

- Chia seeds

- Almond milk

- Mango, pureed

- Agave nectar

- Shredded coconut

Preparation Time: 10 minutes (plus overnight chilling)

Cooking Time: N/A

Serving Time: 15 minutes

Nutritional Info:

- Calories: 160

- Protein: 4g

- Fiber: 8g

- Healthy Fats: 7g

Benefits:

- Chia seeds are a source of Omega-3 fatty acids.

- Mango provides vitamins and antioxidants.

Instructions:

- Mix chia seeds with almond milk, mango puree, and agave nectar.

- Refrigerate overnight.

- Sprinkle with shredded coconut before serving.

Serving Methods:

1. Top with fresh mint leaves for a burst of flavor.

2. Serve as a nutrient-packed dessert or breakfast.

Banana-Oat Cookies

Ingredients:

- Bananas, mashed

- Rolled oats

- Almond butter

- Cinnamon

- Raisins

Preparation Time: 10 minutes

Cooking Time: 15 minutes

Serving Time: 25 minutes

Nutritional Info:

- Calories: 90

- Protein: 3g

- Fiber: 2g

- Healthy Fats: 4g

Benefits:

- Bananas provide potassium and natural sweetness.

- Oats offer soluble fiber.

Instructions:

- Mix mashed bananas with rolled oats, almond butter, cinnamon, and raisins.

- Drop spoonfuls onto a baking sheet and bake until golden.

- Allow to cool before serving.

Serving Methods:

1. Drizzle with a touch of honey for added sweetness.

2. Serve as a wholesome alternative to traditional cookies.

Coconut and Berry Chia Popsicles

Ingredients:

- Coconut milk

- Mixed berries (raspberries, blackberries)

- Chia seeds

- Agave nectar

Preparation Time: 15 minutes (plus freezing)

Cooking Time: N/A

Serving Time: 30 minutes

Nutritional Info:

- Calories: 120

- Protein: 3g

- Fiber: 5g

- Healthy Fats: 8g

Benefits:

- Coconut milk provides healthy fats.

- Berries are rich in antioxidants.

Instructions:

- Blend coconut milk, mixed berries, chia seeds, and agave nectar.

- Pour into popsicle molds and freeze.

- Remove from molds and serve.

Serving Methods:

1. Roll popsicles in shredded coconut before serving.

2. Serve as a refreshing treat on warm days.

Apple and Almond Butter Nachos

Ingredients:

- Apple slices

- Almond butter

- Granola

- Cinnamon

Preparation Time: 10 minutes

Cooking Time: N/A

Serving Time: 15 minutes

Nutritional Info:

- Calories: 110

- Protein: 2g

- Fiber: 3g

- Healthy Fats: 6g

Benefits:

- Apples offer natural sweetness and fiber.

- Almond butter provides healthy fats and protein.

Instructions:

- Arrange apple slices on a plate.

- Drizzle with almond butter and sprinkle with granola and cinnamon.

- Serve immediately.

Serving Methods:

1. Top with a handful of chopped nuts for extra crunch.

2. Serve as a satisfying and nutritious dessert or snack.

Pumpkin Spice Energy Balls

Ingredients:

- Dates, pitted

- Pumpkin puree

- Almond flour

- Pumpkin spice

- Almonds, finely chopped

Preparation Time: 15 minutes

Cooking Time: N/A

Serving Time: 25 minutes

Nutritional Info:

- Calories: 100

- Protein: 3g

- Fiber: 2g

- Healthy Fats: 5g

Benefits:

- Dates provide natural sweetness and fiber.

- Pumpkin is rich in vitamins and antioxidants.

Instructions:

- Blend dates, pumpkin puree, almond flour, and pumpkin spice until a dough forms.

- Roll into small balls and coat with chopped almonds.

- Chill before serving.

Serving Methods:

1. Dust with a sprinkle of extra pumpkin spice before serving.

2. Serve as a convenient energy-boosting dessert.

Almond and Blueberry Frozen Yogurt Bites

Ingredients:

- Greek yogurt

- Almonds, chopped

- Fresh blueberries

- Honey

Preparation Time: 15 minutes (plus freezing)

Cooking Time: N/A

Serving Time: 30 minutes

Nutritional Info:

- Calories: 80

- Protein: 4g

- Fiber: 1g

- Healthy Fats: 3g

Benefits:

- Greek yogurt provides protein and probiotics.

- Blueberries offer antioxidants.

Instructions:

- Mix Greek yogurt with chopped almonds and fresh blueberries.

- Spoon into mini muffin cups and drizzle with honey.

- Freeze until set and serve.

Serving Methods:

1. Garnish with a mint leaf before serving.

2. Serve as bite-sized, cool treats.

Cinnamon Baked Pears

Ingredients:

- Pears, halved

- Cinnamon

- Walnuts, chopped

- Greek yogurt

- Honey

Preparation Time: 15 minutes

Cooking Time: 30 minutes

Serving Time: 45 minutes

Nutritional Info:

- Calories: 130

- Protein: 3g

- Fiber: 5g

- Healthy Fats: 4g

Benefits:

- Pears provide fiber and natural sweetness.

- Walnuts offer Omega-3 fatty acids.

Instructions:

- Preheat the oven to 375°F (190°C).

- Place pear halves on a baking sheet, sprinkle with cinnamon, and top with chopped walnuts.

- Bake until pears are tender.

- Serve with a dollop of Greek yogurt and a drizzle of honey.

Serving Methods:

1. Sprinkle with a pinch of nutmeg before serving.

2. Serve as a warm and comforting dessert.

Dark Chocolate-Dipped Strawberries

Ingredients:

- Fresh strawberries, washed and dried

- Dark chocolate, melted

- Pistachios, finely chopped

- Sea salt

Preparation Time: 15 minutes

Cooking Time: N/A

Serving Time: 20 minutes

Nutritional Info:

- Calories: 90

- Protein: 1g

- Fiber: 2g

- Healthy Fats: 5g

Benefits:

- Dark chocolate provides antioxidants.

- Strawberries are rich in vitamin C.

Instructions:

- Dip each strawberry into melted dark chocolate.

- Sprinkle with chopped pistachios and a pinch of sea salt.

- Place on a parchment-lined tray and allow to set.

Serving Methods:

1. Drizzle with a little honey before serving.

2. Serve as an elegant and indulgent dessert.

Turmeric Golden Milk Popsicles

Ingredients:

- Coconut milk

- Turmeric

- Honey

- Vanilla extract

- Ground cinnamon

Preparation Time: 15 minutes (plus freezing)

Cooking Time: N/A

Serving Time: 30 minutes

Nutritional Info:

- Calories: 100

- Protein: 2g

- Fiber: 1g

- Healthy Fats: 6g

Benefits:

- Turmeric provides anti-inflammatory properties.

- Coconut milk offers healthy fats.

Instructions:

- Mix coconut milk with turmeric, honey, vanilla extract, and ground cinnamon.

- Pour into popsicle molds and freeze until solid.

- Remove from molds and serve.

Serving Methods:

1. Roll popsicles in crushed pistachios before serving.

2. Serve as a refreshing and anti-inflammatory dessert.

Matcha Green Tea Chia Pudding

Ingredients:

- Chia seeds

- Almond milk

- Matcha green tea powder

- Maple syrup

- Fresh berries

Preparation Time: 10 minutes (plus overnight chilling)

Cooking Time: N/A

Serving Time: 15 minutes

Nutritional Info:

- Calories: 120

- Protein: 4g

- Fiber: 6g

- Healthy Fats: 5g

Benefits:

- Matcha is rich in antioxidants and promotes relaxation.

- Chia seeds provide Omega-3 fatty acids.

Instructions:

- Mix chia seeds with almond milk, matcha powder, and maple syrup.

- Refrigerate overnight.

- Top with fresh berries before serving.

Serving Methods:

1. Garnish with a mint leaf for a burst of freshness.

2. Serve as a nutrient-packed dessert or breakfast.

Papaya and Lime Sorbet

Ingredients:

- Ripe papaya, diced

- Lime juice

- Agave nectar

- Fresh mint leaves

Preparation Time: 15 minutes (plus freezing)

Cooking Time: N/A

Serving Time: 30 minutes

Nutritional Info:

- Calories: 80

- Protein: 1g

- Fiber: 2g

- Healthy Fats: 0g

Benefits:

- Papaya provides digestive enzymes and vitamins.

- Lime juice offers a burst of vitamin C.

Instructions:

- Blend diced papaya with lime juice and agave nectar.

- Pour into a shallow dish and freeze.

- Scoop into bowls and garnish with fresh mint leaves.

Serving Methods:

1. Drizzle with a touch of chili powder for a hint of spice.

2. Serve as a tropical and refreshing dessert.

Walnut and Date Energy Bites

Ingredients:

- Dates, pitted

- Walnuts

- Unsweetened shredded coconut

- Vanilla extract

- Ground flaxseeds

Preparation Time: 15 minutes

Cooking Time: N/A

Serving Time: 25 minutes

Nutritional Info:

- Calories: 90

- Protein: 2g

- Fiber: 2g

- Healthy Fats: 5g

Benefits:

- Dates provide natural sweetness and fiber.

- Walnuts offer Omega-3 fatty acids.

Instructions:

- Blend dates, walnuts, shredded coconut, vanilla extract, and ground flaxseeds.

- Roll into small balls and chill before serving.

Serving Methods:

1. Coat with a thin layer of dark chocolate for added richness.

2. Serve as a convenient and wholesome energy-boosting dessert.

Blueberry and Almond Flour Mug Cake

Ingredients:

- Almond flour

- Blueberries

- Maple syrup

- Baking powder

- Almond milk

Preparation Time: 10 minutes

Cooking Time: 5 minutes

Serving Time: 15 minutes

Nutritional Info:

- Calories: 120

- Protein: 4g

- Fiber: 3g

- Healthy Fats: 6g

Benefits:

- Almond flour provides a gluten-free alternative.

- Blueberries offer antioxidants.

Instructions:

- Mix almond flour, blueberries, maple syrup, baking powder, and almond milk in a mug.

- Microwave until set.

- Allow to cool slightly before serving.

Serving Methods:

1. Top with a dollop of coconut whipped cream.

2. Serve as a warm and comforting single-serving dessert.

Cocoa Avocado Pudding

Ingredients:

- Ripe avocados

- Cocoa powder

- Almond milk

- Honey

- Chopped pistachios

Preparation Time: 15 minutes

Cooking Time: N/A

Serving Time: 30 minutes

Nutritional Info:

- Calories: 150

- Protein: 3g

- Fiber: 5g

- Healthy Fats: 10g

Benefits:

- Avocados provide creamy texture and healthy fats.

- Cocoa powder is rich in antioxidants.

Instructions:

- Blend avocados, cocoa powder, almond milk, and honey until smooth.

- Chill in the refrigerator.

- Garnish with chopped pistachios before serving.

Serving Methods:

1. Sprinkle with a pinch of sea salt for a sweet-savory contrast.

2. Serve as a decadent and nutrient-packed chocolate pudding.

Raspberry and Almond Tartlets

Ingredients:

- Almond flour tartlet shells

- Greek yogurt

- Fresh raspberries

- Agave nectar

- Sliced almonds

Preparation Time: 20 minutes

Cooking Time: 10 minutes

Serving Time: 30 minutes

Nutritional Info:

- Calories: 110

- Protein: 4g

- Fiber: 2g

- Healthy Fats: 6g

Benefits:

- Almond flour provides a gluten-free crust.

- Raspberries offer antioxidants and vitamins.

Instructions:

- Fill almond flour tartlet shells with Greek yogurt.

- Top with fresh raspberries and drizzle with agave nectar.

- Sprinkle sliced almonds before serving.

Serving Methods:

1. Dust with a light layer of powdered cinnamon before serving.

2. Serve as a visually appealing and fruity dessert.

Coconut and Pineapple Chia Seed Popsicles

Ingredients:

- Coconut water

- Chia seeds

- Pineapple chunks

- Coconut flakes

Preparation Time: 15 minutes (plus freezing)

Cooking Time: N/A

Serving Time: 30 minutes

Nutritional Info:

- Calories: 80

- Protein: 2g

- Fiber: 4g

- Healthy Fats: 3g

Benefits:

- Chia seeds provide Omega-3 fatty acids.

- Coconut water is hydrating and refreshing.

Instructions:

- Mix coconut water with chia seeds and pineapple chunks.

- Pour into popsicle molds and freeze until solid.

- Roll popsicles in coconut flakes before serving.

Serving Methods:

1. Drizzle with a touch of lime juice for a tropical twist.

2. Serve as a hydrating and wholesome dessert.

Pomegranate and Pistachio Frozen Yogurt Bites

Ingredients:

- Greek yogurt

- Pomegranate seeds

- Pistachios, chopped

- Maple syrup

Preparation Time: 15 minutes (plus freezing)

Cooking Time: N/A

Serving Time: 30 minutes

Nutritional Info:

- Calories: 70

- Protein: 3g

- Fiber: 1g

- Healthy Fats: 2g

Benefits:

- Pomegranate seeds offer antioxidants.

- Greek yogurt provides protein and probiotics.

Instructions:

- Mix Greek yogurt with pomegranate seeds, chopped pistachios, and maple syrup.

- Spoon into mini muffin cups and freeze until set.

- Serve chilled.

Serving Methods:

1. Garnish with a sprinkle of crushed mint leaves before serving.

2. Serve as a bite-sized and cool treat.

Mango and Coconut Rice Pudding

Ingredients:

- Arborio rice

- Coconut milk

- Fresh mango, diced

- Agave nectar

- Toasted coconut flakes

Preparation Time: 20 minutes

Cooking Time: 30 minutes

Serving Time: 50 minutes

Nutritional Info:

- Calories: 130

- Protein: 2g

- Fiber: 1g

- Healthy Fats: 5g

Benefits:

- Coconut milk provides a creamy texture.

- Mango offers vitamins and natural sweetness.

Instructions:

- Cook Arborio rice in coconut milk until creamy.

- Sweeten with agave nectar and fold in diced mango.

- Chill before serving and garnish with toasted coconut flakes.

Serving Methods:

1. Sprinkle with a pinch of ground cardamom before serving.

2. Serve as a tropical and satisfying rice pudding

CHAPTER EIGHT
MEAL PLAN

Day 1

- **Breakfast:** Berry Yogurt Parfait

- **Lunch:** Quinoa and Vegetable Stuffed Bell Peppers

- **Snack:** Walnut and Date Energy Bites

- **Dinner:** Coconut and Berry Chia Popsicles

- **Dessert:** Turmeric Golden Milk Popsicles

Day 2

- **Breakfast:** Matcha Green Tea Chia Pudding

- **Lunch:** Smoked Salmon Cucumber Bites

- **Snack:** Blueberry and Almond Flour Mug Cake

- **Dinner:** Walnut and Date Energy Bites

- **Dessert:** Cocoa Avocado Pudding

Day 3

- **Breakfast:** Papaya and Lime Sorbet

- **Lunch:** Zucchini and Goat Cheese Roll-Ups

- **Snack:** Raspberry and Almond Tartlets

- **Dinner:** Pumpkin Spice Energy Balls

- **Dessert:** Walnut and Date Energy Bites

Day 4

- **Breakfast:** Banana-Oat Cookies

- **Lunch:** Tuna Salad Lettuce Wraps

- **Snack:** Cinnamon Baked Pears

- **Dinner:** Cauliflower Buffalo Bites

- **Dessert:** Dark Chocolate-Dipped Strawberries

Day 5

- **Breakfast:** Chia Seed and Mango Pudding

- **Lunch:** Mushroom and Spinach Stuffed Phyllo Cups

- **Snack:** Apple and Almond Butter Nachos

- **Dinner:** Egg Salad Stuffed Cucumber Cups

- **Dessert:** Coconut and Pineapple Chia Seed Popsicles

Day 6

- **Breakfast:** Greek Yogurt with Fresh Fruit

- **Lunch:** Caprese Skewers

- **Snack:** Sesame Ginger Snap Peas

- **Dinner:** Guacamole-Stuffed Cucumber Cups

- **Dessert:** Pomegranate and Pistachio Frozen Yogurt Bites

Day 7

- **Breakfast:** Avocado Toast with Tomato Slices

- **Lunch:** Guacamole-Stuffed Cucumber Cups

- **Snack:** Quinoa and Vegetable Stuffed Bell Peppers

- **Dinner:** Zucchini and Goat Cheese Roll-Ups

- **Dessert:** Mango and Coconut Rice Pudding

Day 8

- **Breakfast:** Greek Yogurt with Fresh Fruit

- **Lunch:** Caprese Skewers

- **Snack:** Sesame Ginger Snap Peas

- **Dinner:** Guacamole-Stuffed Cucumber Cups

- **Dessert:** Pomegranate and Pistachio Frozen Yogurt Bites

Day 9

- **Breakfast:** Avocado Toast with Tomato Slices

- **Lunch:** Guacamole-Stuffed Cucumber Cups

- **Snack:** Quinoa and Vegetable Stuffed Bell Peppers

- **Dinner:** Zucchini and Goat Cheese Roll-Ups

- **Dessert:** Mango and Coconut Rice Pudding

Day 10

- **Breakfast:** Berry Yogurt Parfait

- **Lunch:** Quinoa and Vegetable Stuffed Bell Peppers

- **Snack:** Walnut and Date Energy Bites

- **Dinner:** Coconut and Berry Chia Popsicles

- **Dessert:** Turmeric Golden Milk Popsicles

Day 11

- **Breakfast:** Matcha Green Tea Chia Pudding

- **Lunch:** Smoked Salmon Cucumber Bites

- **Snack:** Blueberry and Almond Flour Mug Cake

- **Dinner:** Walnut and Date Energy Bites

- **Dessert:** Cocoa Avocado Pudding

Day 12

- **Breakfast:** Papaya and Lime Sorbet

- **Lunch:** Zucchini and Goat Cheese Roll-Ups

- **Snack:** Raspberry and Almond Tartlets

- **Dinner:** Pumpkin Spice Energy Balls

- **Dessert:** Walnut and Date Energy Bites

Day 13

- **Breakfast:** Banana-Oat Cookies

- **Lunch:** Tuna Salad Lettuce Wraps

- **Snack:** Cinnamon Baked Pears

- **Dinner:** Cauliflower Buffalo Bites

- **Dessert:** Dark Chocolate-Dipped Strawberries

Day 14

- **Breakfast:** Chia Seed and Mango Pudding

- **Lunch:** Mushroom and Spinach Stuffed Phyllo Cups

- **Snack:** Apple and Almond Butter Nachos

- **Dinner:** Egg Salad Stuffed Cucumber Cups

- **Dessert:** Coconut and Pineapple Chia Seed Popsicles

Day 15

- **Breakfast:** Matcha Green Tea Chia Pudding

- **Lunch:** Smoked Salmon Cucumber Bites

- **Snack:** Blueberry and Almond Flour Mug Cake

- **Dinner:** Walnut and Date Energy Bites

- **Dessert:** Cocoa Avocado Pudding

Day 16

- **Breakfast:** Papaya and Lime Sorbet

- **Lunch:** Zucchini and Goat Cheese Roll-Ups

- **Snack:** Raspberry and Almond Tartlets

- **Dinner:** Pumpkin Spice Energy Balls

- **Dessert:** Walnut and Date Energy Bites

Day 17

- **Breakfast:** Banana-Oat Cookies
- **Lunch:** Tuna Salad Lettuce Wraps
- **Snack:** Cinnamon Baked Pears
- **Dinner:** Cauliflower Buffalo Bites
- **Dessert:** Dark Chocolate-Dipped Strawberries

Day 18

- **Breakfast:** Greek Yogurt with Fresh Fruit
- **Lunch:** Caprese Skewers
- **Snack:** Sesame Ginger Snap Peas
- **Dinner:** Guacamole-Stuffed Cucumber Cups
- **Dessert:** Pomegranate and Pistachio Frozen Yogurt Bites

Day 19

- **Breakfast:** Avocado Toast with Tomato Slices
- **Lunch:** Guacamole-Stuffed Cucumber Cups
- **Snack:** Quinoa and Vegetable Stuffed Bell Peppers
- **Dinner:** Zucchini and Goat Cheese Roll-Ups

- **Dessert:** Mango and Coconut Rice Pudding

Day 20

- **Breakfast:** Chia Seed and Mango Pudding

- **Lunch:** Mushroom and Spinach Stuffed Phyllo Cups

- **Snack:** Apple and Almond Butter Nachos

- **Dinner:** Egg Salad Stuffed Cucumber Cups

- **Dessert:** Coconut and Pineapple Chia Seed Popsicles

Day 21

- **Breakfast:** Berry Yogurt Parfait

- **Lunch:** Quinoa and Vegetable Stuffed Bell Peppers

- **Snack:** Walnut and Date Energy Bites

- **Dinner:** Coconut and Berry Chia Popsicles

- **Dessert:** Turmeric Golden Milk Popsicles

CONCLUSION

In conclusion, the Alzheimer's Diet Cookbook for Beginners offers a holistic approach to supporting brain health through nutrition. Throughout this book, we have explored the fundamentals of Alzheimer's disease, the impact of nutrition on cognitive function, and the importance of a balanced diet in managing its symptoms. By focusing on key nutrients for brain health and providing practical guidelines for setting up an Alzheimer's-friendly kitchen, this cookbook empowers readers to make informed dietary choices.

From nutritious breakfast options like the Berry Yogurt Parfait to satisfying dinner recipes like the Egg Salad Stuffed Cucumber Cups, each dish is thoughtfully crafted to provide essential nutrients while catering to the taste preferences of individuals with Alzheimer's and their caregivers. Additionally, the inclusion of snacks and appetizers such as the Sesame Ginger Snap Peas and Walnut and Date Energy Bites offers convenient and delicious options to maintain energy levels throughout the day.

The dessert section introduces indulgent yet nutritious treats like the Cocoa Avocado Pudding and the Coconut and Pineapple Chia Seed Popsicles, showcasing that healthy eating can still be enjoyable and flavorful. Moreover, the provided 21-day meal plan offers a structured approach to incorporating these recipes into daily life, promoting consistency and variety in dietary choices.

Overall, this cookbook serves as a valuable resource for individuals navigating the challenges of Alzheimer's disease and seeking practical strategies to support brain health through nutrition. By emphasizing the importance of a nutrient-rich diet and providing a diverse range of recipes, the Alzheimer's Diet Cookbook for Beginners empowers readers to take proactive steps towards improving their overall well-being and quality of life.